Providing **Practice**

Fourth edition

Comments and reviews of earlier editions of
Providing Diabetes Care in General Practice:

'The complete guide for the primary health care team.' – Dr Michael Hall,
Chairman, Diabetes UK

'It is a real contribution to a modern understanding of so many aspects of
diabetes.' – Professor Harry Keen, former Vice President, Diabetes UK

'An extremely useful text for primary healthcare teams in improving the quality
of care for people with diabetes.' – Dr John Toby, Chairman of Joint
Committee, Royal College of General Practitioners

'Anyone reading it will be in very safe hands and feel their confidence in
diabetes growing chapter by chapter.' – Dr Charles Fox, Consultant Physician,
Northampton General Hospital

'The book has been invaluable, specifically in helping us set up our training
practices in diabetes and the courses attached to this scheme.' – Helma Grant,
Practice Nurse, Leicestershire

'I think the book is even better than ever.' – Gwen Hall, Practice Nurse, Surrey

'I love the practical approach taken in the book . . . which I am sure will help
primary care practitioners save time and produce a better service.' – Dr Charles
Price, Consultant in Public Health Medicine, Sheffield Health

'The book is an extraordinary and necessary piece of information.' – Maria L de
Alva, former President, International Diabetes Federation

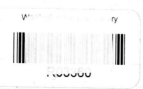

Dedication

For people with diabetes and those who care for them.

To Ewen, Alastair and Duncan:
For their love and support.

To Margaret Haynes, Practice Nurse:
Carterknowle Road and Dore Medical Practice, Sheffield
For her compassion, for listening and for looking after me so well.

About the author

Mary MacKinnon MMed Sci, RGN was appointed Senior Lecturer in Diabetes Care at the University of Warwick in 1999, and is the Director of Education for Warwick Diabetes Care, which was launched in November 2000.

Mary was Diabetes Services Co-ordinator and University Lecturer in Sheffield between 1987 and 1999. From 1997 to 1999 she was seconded as Consultant to Diabetes UK (formerly the British Diabetic Association) to facilitate the setting up of a new professional section, Primary Care Diabetes UK (PCDUK). She is currently PCDUK Honorary Secretary.

For 17 years, Mary has worked in diabetes care in Sheffield as a practice nurse, diabetes researcher, facilitator and educator. She has written/co-written books on diabetes for the primary care team, writing extensively on the subject and other aspects of diabetes care and education. She was a member of the BDA/DoH Joint Task Force for Diabetes and has been involved in the work of two subgroups for the National Service Framework for Diabetes.

Mary has worked for the International Diabetes Federation (IDF) over a number of years. She was an IDF Vice-President 1994–1997 and an officer of the IDF Diabetes Education Consultative Section 1994–2000.

She now has type 2 diabetes.

Providing Diabetes Care in General Practice

A Practical Guide to Integrated Care

Fourth edition

Mary MacKinnon MMed Sci, RGN

Senior Lecturer in Diabetes Care and Director of Education,
Warwick Diabetes Care, University of Warwick, Coventry, UK

Class Publishing • London

First edition, 1993
Second edition, 1995
Third edition, 1998
Fourth edition, 2002

A CIP catalogue record for this book is available from the British Library

ISBN 1 85959 048 9

The author and publishers welcome feedback from the users of this book.

Class Publishing, Barb House, Barb Mews, London W6 7PA, UK
email: post@class.co.uk
website: www.class.co.uk

Designed and typeset by Martin Bristow

Printed and bound in Slovenia by Mladisnka knjiga,
by arrangement with Korotan, Ljubljana

Contents

Foreword

Michael Hall

I welcome this new edition of *Providing Diabetes Care in General Practice*, which represents an updated guide for the primary health care team. Its appearance, as the National Service Framework for Diabetes is about to be published, is timely.

The whole world is faced with increasing numbers of people with diabetes and, largely because of effective interventions, the expectation is that those afflicted should enjoy a long life and a healthy lifestyle. As a consequence, there are not only increased numbers of people with diabetes, but also increased numbers of people with the complications of the condition. It has become a real challenge for the primary care team.

There is a new feeling of excitement and vitality about in the health service, nowhere more so than in diabetes care. There are new opportunities that can improve quality of life and reduce the risk of complications of diabetes.

We know that successful management depends on good glycaemic and blood pressure control and detection of the earliest signs of complications. Studies have shown that helping those with diabetes to achieve a greater understanding of their condition is very important to improving good control, while at the same time minimising the impact of diabetes on their quality of life. Part of this book is about helping professionals to provide a good education in diabetes to their patients and thus empowering patients to take greater responsibility for their own management.

Providing a regular surveillance service for all those with diabetes is an accepted part of the role of the health care team. The difficulty of keeping track of so many people through hospital-based services, especially when so many people with diabetes rarely attend hospital, is well known. It is now possible to set up local diabetes registers linked with the population registers of general practitioners. These can provide the opportunity for monitoring individuals as well as being a valuable tool to assist in auditing the local diabetes service.

New arrangements for diabetes care in general practice have taken account of the best professional advice in both specialist and primary care. It will allow GPs, practice nurses and other professionals in the primary health care teams to link with expert resources, such as diabetes specialist nurses, and to become central players in diabetes care.

I welcome this book which will help all those wishing to plan or participate in a diabetes care programme. The well-referenced index makes it quick and easy to use.

Dr Michael Hall
General Practitioner
Chairman, Diabetes UK

Foreword

Colin Kenny

Francis Bacon said that 'some books are to be tasted, others to be swallowed, and some few to be chewed and digested'. I am pleased to see a fourth edition of *Providing Diabetes Care in General Practice* because I have chewed and digested much of my current edition. It has been used continually to answer questions from patients and to prepare articles and talks, as well as being a general reference text.

This fourth edition is very welcome because it details many of the contemporary changes in general practice and primary diabetes care. The 1990s was a decade of change for the management of diabetes, with the balance of routine diabetes care being actively commissioned by general practitioners. This shift to primary care management has been accompanied by an overall change in focus for the NHS, with the introduction of evidence-based medicine, clinical governance and National Service Frameworks. Many of these changes are acknowledged in this new edition.

Mary MacKinnon was also instrumental in initiating a separate voice for Primary Care Diabetes. Primary Care Diabetes UK (PCDUK) is now a full section of the revamped Diabetes UK. It caters for all those caring for people with diabetes in this expanding primary care sector. This organisation represents all those involved in this aspect of primary care, as well as advocating high-quality patient care. The aims are encapsulated in the group's mission statement:

> Encouraging high quality and culturally sensitive care for people with diabetes within primary care.

People with diabetes in primary care are a different, and much larger, subset from those seen in hospital. They are often older and frequently disadvantaged. One of the strengths of primary care is not to take either diseases or patients in isolation, but to see them as part of larger family groups, and the wider community.

The problems and challenges of high-quality diabetes care continue. Diabetes mellitus is set to become a significant twenty-first century problem. We know that already up to 10% of the NHS budget may be devoted to diabetes care, with long-term chronic illness forming a significant portion of this. The evidence-based United Kingdom Prospective Diabetes Study (UKPDS) demonstrated that the intensive management of blood glucose concentration and hypertension reduces the risk of complications in patients with type 2 diabetes. This presents primary care with a considerable challenge. Worldwide, it is estimated that the number of people with diabetes will double within the next 10 years, putting a significant strain on all health care systems.

The fourth edition of this very accessible textbook offers the reader a very useful overview of the problems associated with having diabetes, as well as suggesting models for care. I would recommend it to any member of the diabetes care team wishing to improve their standards of care.

Dr Colin Kenny
General Practitioner
Formerly Chairman, Primary Care Diabetes UK

Diabetes care in the UK: progress since the St Vincent Declaration

Harry Keen, Vice-President (former Chairman), British Diabetic Association; Honorary President, International Diabetes Federation

In the foreword to the first edition of this book, I drew attention to the UK response to the 1989 St Vincent Declaration on Diabetes. This milestone Declaration was essentially a call to action from the European Offices of the World Health Organization and of the International Diabetes Federation. The Declaration was put together at a unique meeting of people with diabetes, their care providers, representatives from almost all European government health departments, the pharmaceutical industry and the media. It set out, in a one-page document, a series of quite specific objectives which, if achieved, would notably improve the prospects for life and health of people with diabetes.

The Declaration included a number of ambitious quantitative targets: to reduce retinopathic blindness, diabetic renal failure, lower limb amputations, pregnancy loss and birth defects, and the great burden of heart disease and stroke. These targets were tough but achievable. Every European society, how-ever rich or poor, could anticipate a rise in the size of the personal, social and economic burdens of diabetes and its complications. They could all move towards substantial reductions in these burdens by improving and modernising their diabetes care. But only professional determination, political will and the pressure of people with diabetes themselves could convert the aspirations of the Declaration into reality.

In response to the Declaration, the UK set up a Joint British Diabetic Association (BDA; now Diabetes UK)/Department of Health St Vincent Task Force for Diabetes. Under the chairmanship of Professor David Shaw, it included doctors and nurses from specialist units and primary care, representatives of management, government and the Health Departments of Scotland, Northern Ireland and Wales, and people with diabetes themselves. The Task Force drew upon countrywide expertise, setting up 11 Expert Advisory Subgroups covering the following subjects and their comprehensive reports were published in a sup-plement to *Diabetic Medicine*:

- information
- visual disability
- renal disease
- diabetic foot and amputation

- children and young people
- pregnancy and neonatal
- patients and carers
- research and development
- professional training
- clinical care
- cardiovascular disease.

The Task Force visited many localities and handed its final Report and Recommendations to Ministers and to the BDA, both of whom accepted it with enthusiasm. Problems arose with implementation but eventually a document called 'Key Features of a Good Diabetes Service' was prepared and distributed as guidance to all health authorities and trusts. In the meantime the BDA had taken a lead, stimulating the organisation of Local Diabetes Services Advisory Groups with over 150 of them around the country.

All of this was against the background of major changes in the pattern of diabetes care provision in the NHS. Primary care has become a major agent in the organisation and provision of systematic diabetes care to their patients. Increasingly, the local Diabetes Specialist Group is acting as a resource and support for primary care colleagues. A most important recent change was the decision of the Department of Health to create a National Service Framework (NSF) for Diabetes. The purpose of this NSF is to ensure accessibility to high standards of modern diabetes care right across the country, building upon the strong foundation created by the St Vincent Declaration. Like the Joint Task Force, the NSF has brought together all the stakeholders in diabetes care and, at the time of writing, we await its Report and Recommendations which, we are assured, will be adequately resourced. When it goes into action as expected in 2002, it will greatly reinforce the pursuit of the great St Vincent aims by bringing the best of modern practice to people with diabetes right across the country.

But make no mistake. The NSF is just the beginning of a process that will make increased demands on all those concerned with diabetes care. The professionals will need to update their knowledge and training. People with diabetes, major care providers themselves, will need to contribute and collaborate actively. NHS management must throw itself wholeheartedly into the implementation process, seeking new and innovative ways to deliver the goods. The next few years can be most exciting and fulfilling for people with diabetes, lifting the threats of ill health and improving the quality of life. But this will become a reality only with the active, sustained and cooperative effort of many hundreds of thousands of people who know what they do – and do what they know!

Further reading

British Diabetic Association (1995). *Guidance for Local Diabetes Services Advisory Groups.* London: BDA.

Department of Health/British Diabetic Association (1995). *Report of the St Vincent Joint Task Force for Diabetes.* London: BDA.

Specialist Workgroup Reports (1996). St Vincent and improving diabetes care. *Diabetic Medicine* **13** (suppl 4).

Living with diabetes: my story

Dear Colleagues,

In March 1999, in Yaounde, Cameroon, while facilitating a diabetes leadership course for health care professionals in Africa, I found I had diabetes. This discovery was made as I tested my own blood glucose using a new meter and strips, alongside the course participants, who were doing likewise. The blood glucose level reading was 15 mmol/l and I quickly closed the device, so as to hide the result from my colleagues. This ploy backfired as another member of the teaching faculty opened the meter, which memorised the last test made!

I decided to tell the course participants the result of the blood glucose test and ask them to prepare a plan of diabetes management for me, which they duly did. I also informed them that I had felt unwell for several months but had put this down to the aftermath of a very severe bout of flu. I had in fact felt exhausted for some time and latterly had been thirstier than usual and prone to frequent infections. The course members produced textbook management plans and I learned how irrelevant these are when you are newly diagnosed and when disbelief, fear and denial may prevail over all else. When one of the people in the room took me aside, put his arm around me and asked me how I was feeling, I learned how important real empathy is at such a time.

We now have greater knowledge of the impact of the diagnosis from research evidence and from the narrative of personal experience of people with diabetes. However, I was not prepared for the effect of discovering I had the condition, nor the impact that this had on my family who, like myself, were disbelieving and devastated by the news.

Once the diagnosis was confirmed and with all good intentions, I set out to follow the conventional treatment protocol of reviewing and making changes to my diet, reducing my food intake, walking the dog much more and paid up to join a fitness centre. Within two weeks, I had a stress fracture in my left foot and the dog was begging for mercy! At around six weeks, following the confirmation of the diagnosis, I had lost a little weight but remained very tired, lethargic and thirsty and, in discussion with my family doctor, started on the lowest dose of metformin. My experience with the minimum dose of this drug lasted for several months and would fill another book! Like 30% of those who embark on metformin therapy, I had to abandon it and, in my case, begin the sulphonylurea trail.

So my journey with diabetes continues. Even though I know a little about this condition, I continually learn something new about living with diabetes and about other people's attitudes to it and to me, every day. I remain an individual with many weaknesses and understand how it feels to fail, to feel guilty when I fail and to be judged by others. I know how difficult it is to do what you ought to do every day.

During the long year following my diagnosis, I appreciated so much the love of my family and the wonderful support from the doctors and, especially, the practice nurse at our local surgery, who know us and have looked after us for over 20 years.

It is because of them that I am able to do my work at Warwick Diabetes Care. Perhaps I should also let you know that, although I joined a fitness centre, I haven't actually been to it yet!

I wish you well in your important work in helping people with diabetes to look after themselves. Please remember that it is not easy for them to do this and your vital role is to support them in their endeavours. Caring for a person with diabetes is not just about achieving perfect laboratory results or government targets, it is much, much more and is encompassed in this gentle reminder:

> Don't walk in front of me
> I may not follow.
> Don't walk behind me
> I may not lead.
> Walk beside me
> and
> Just be my friend.

Best wishes,

Mary MacKinnon
Senior Lecturer, University of Warwick
Director of Education, Warwick Diabetes Care

August 2001

Acknowledgements

I would like to take this opportunity to thank certain special people who have advised or contributed to the fourth edition, at the same time acknowledging those similarly involved in previous editions. They have, with kindness and generosity, given valuable time to the book. My grateful thanks go to them all.

Fourth edition
Dr Michael Hall – General Practitioner and Chairman, Diabetes UK
Professor Harry Keen – former Vice-President, Diabetes UK
Dr Colin Kenny – General Practitioner and first Chairman, Primary Care Diabetes UK
Mrs Jane Sugarman – Editing Consultant
Mrs Louise Dodd – Practice Nurse and Diabetes Research Co-ordinator, University of Warwick
Dr Charles Fox – Consultant Physician, Northampton General Hospital
Dr Roger Gadsby – General Practitioner and Medical Director, Warwick Diabetes Care, University of Warwick
Mrs Surinder Ghatoray – Community Dietitian and Senior Teaching Fellow, Warwick Diabetes Care, University of Warwick
Mrs Julia Gilroy – Diabetes Specialist Nurse and Diabetes Lead Nurse, North Solihull Health
Dr Vinod Patel – Consultant Physician, George Eliot Hospital, Nuneaton
Dr Mohan Pawa – General Practitioner and Vice-Chairman, Primary Care Diabetes UK

Previous editions
Dr Charles Fox, Ms Helma Grant, Mrs Gwen Hall, Dr Simon Heller, Dr Norman How, Dr Eugene Hughes, Ms Katherine Kennedy, Dr Alastair Mackie, Ms Judith North, Ms Jill Rogers, Dr Jenny Stephenson and Ms Ruth Webber.

Introduction

This fourth edition will be available in a new millennium and at the dawn of a new era in health care for people with diabetes and 'those who care for them' in the United Kingdom. In 2002, the implementation of a National Service Framework for Diabetes (England and Wales) will begin. A National Framework for Scotland is planned within a similar timescale.

The purpose of this book is to provide a practical, helpful and up-to-date guide to the integrated care of people with diabetes in the primary care setting, with the aim of reducing known variations in diabetes services and raising standards of health care overall. This is the main purpose of the proposed National Service Framework for Diabetes.

The book aims to be of use to all those involved in providing diabetes care. It is set out for easy use in the working situation and is divided into three parts.

Part I: Diabetes – an overview
This sets the scene and includes the roles and educational needs of the primary care team in providing person-centred integrated diabetes care. This care will be delivered in the context of the proposed National Service Framework for Diabetes in line with the modernisation of the NHS set out in *The NHS Plan*.

Part II: Providing diabetes care
This describes how to set up and run a diabetes service in the setting of general practice.

Part III: About diabetes
This provides further information about the disease and its associated complications.

Further information about the condition relating to guidelines and recommendations is included in the Appendices. Throughout the book, summaries are used for quick reference.

Diabetes mellitus: setting the scene in 2001

Over the last decade, there has been a leap in the availability and quality of information technology and in our understanding of diabetes health care and its costs. Research evidence has given us new insights into the management of the disease. Continuing and relentless research and development into new therapies, technologies, quality-of-life measurement and health care organisation and delivery require us to keep up to date and acquire new skills, more than ever before. All health care professionals providing diabetes care have a responsibility to keep up to date and to provide people with diabetes in their care with up-to-date information. For those working in primary care, there is a Diabetes UK professional section (PCDUK) for them to join. More information can be found in Appendix IV.

The global situation

In 2000, new World Health Organization (WHO) criteria for the classification and diagnosis of diabetes were published. Levels for the diagnosis of diabetes were lowered, thereby increasing the burden of the disease. In addition, there is clear evidence of the predicted increasing prevalence of diabetes worldwide in developed and developing countries. The 1998 WHO Report, *World Health*, presents the following facts:

- Diabetes cases in adults will more than double globally from 143 million in 1997 to 300 million in 2025 as a result of population growth, ageing and urbanisation.
- The rising prevalence of diabetes mellitus is closely associated in much of the developing world with industrialisation and socioeconomic development.
- WHO estimates that, of 143 million people affected by diabetes in 1997, 63% were resident in developing countries. By 2025, this proportion will rise to 76%.
- In 1997 and 2025, the three countries with the largest number of people with diabetes are and will be China, India and the USA.
- Whereas, in developed countries, the greatest number of people with diabetes are aged 65 years and above, in developing countries most are aged between 45 and 64. This tendency is expected to accentuate by 2025.
- In developing countries, increasingly people will be affected by diabetes in the most productive period of their lives.
- People developing diabetes at an earlier age have longer in which to develop the long-term complications, such as blindness, kidney failure and heart disease.

New research and developments in diabetes

United Kingdom Prospective Study (UKPDS 1998)

In the last 5 years and particularly since the third edition of this book was published in the spring 1998, new insights and knowledge have emerged. The results of the most extensive trial in type 2 diabetes, the United Kingdom Prospective Diabetes Study (UKPDS), were announced at the European Association Study of Diabetes (EASD) Congress in Barcelona in September 1998. UKPDS results provided strong evidence that type 2 diabetes is a complex metabolic disorder with high risks for cardiovascular disease. The study demonstrated that long-term complications of diabetes could be reduced with intensive strategies for the treatment of hypertension and hyperglycaemia. More information and references can be found in Chapter 22.

Prevalence and incidence of type 2 diabetes (Poole 1998)

The Poole Study identified that over 100,000 people are diagnosed each year in the UK and that the number of cases among men is significantly higher than among women, a marked shift from the position 20–30 years earlier when the reverse was true. More information and references can be found in Chapters 5 and 22.

New classification and diagnosis of diabetes (1998–2001)

New criteria for the identification of those at risk of diabetes and for the diagnosis of the condition followed revision and recommendations by the American Diabetes Association (ADA). These were endorsed by the WHO after consultation. Both groups have lowered the fasting blood glucose (FBG) cut-off from 7.8 mmol/l to 7.0 mmol/l, thereby identifying diabetes at an earlier stage. More information and references can be found in Chapter 5.

The Hypertension Optimal Treatment (HOT) Study (1998)

This large study of older people was designed to investigate the optimum target level for diastolic blood pressure. Results showed a marked reduction in cardiovascular events when the target for diastolic blood pressure was reduced from 90 mmHg to 80 mmHg. More information and references can be found in Chapter 22.

Primary Care Diabetes – a National Enquiry (2000)

A National Enquiry in England and Wales supported by Diabetes UK (formerly the British Diabetic Association) confirmed that, over the past decade, the focus of diabetes care has shifted. Results showed that most diabetes care is provided in general practice (confirming the Audit Commission findings), although there are significant geographical variations in the delivery of primary diabetes care. More information and references can be found in Chapter 22.

New therapies, technology and self-care programmes in diabetes

New oral hypoglycaemic agents as well as new insulin therapies have become licensed and are available. Islet cell transplantation and inhaled insulin are being developed further in efforts to reduce the treatment burden of diabetes. For those with type 1 diabetes, a self-care structured education programme (DAFNE), where people with diabetes learn to match their carbohydrate intake and activity with precise insulin dose adjustments, although still in the research stage, shows promising results. New technology is available where digital imaging for retinal screening is now possible and at a lower cost. Technological progress in the form of non-invasive glucose sensors is being made in the area of blood glucose monitoring.

Changes in the National Health Service

Primary care

The NHS Plan presented in 2000 follows other government papers introducing the greatest changes, particularly in primary care, in the National Health Service since its inception in 1945. These changes have included the introduction of Primary Care Groups (Local Health Care Co-operatives in Scotland and Local Care Groups in Wales). These groups encompass general practices in a locality and cover the primary health care provision to populations of 50,000 up to 150,000. The commissioning role of Health Authorities is gradually devolving to Primary Care Groups, which are now merging to form Primary Care Trusts, covering larger populations.

Clinical governance

Clinical governance has been introduced in all clinical settings in the NHS to ensure that evidence-based standards of care are met, health care professionals are able to put evidence-based care into practice, and systems of audit and quality improvement are visible and monitored. For this to happen, a lead person is accountable for clinical governance in every NHS care organisation and a strategy for the progress of information technology in the NHS is in place for implementation over the next 10 years.

The NHS Plan

In *The NHS Plan* is a 5-year plan for investment and reform and includes sustained increases in funding to enable far-reaching changes throughout the NHS to be achieved. National Service Frameworks for Mental Health, Coronary Heart Disease, Older People and the NHS Cancer Plan are in the public domain. By the spring in 2002, the National Service Framework for Diabetes will also be available and at the first stage of implementation.

Audit Commission Report 2000 – 'Testing Times': a review of diabetes services in England and Wales

Published in April 2000, the Audit Commission Report – *Testing Times* – highlighted variations in specialist diabetes services in nine health districts in England and Wales.

The real experiences and views of people with diabetes and their carers were also sought and featured as 'snapshots' throughout the Report. People with diabetes were found to be dissatisfied with the amount of time health care professionals could spend with them. The poor understanding of diabetes by large numbers of people with the condition, particularly those among certain ethnic groups, was revealed and highlighted in the Report.

Health authorities and general practitioners were also surveyed by post. The postal survey in general practice indicated the extent of diabetes care provided or part provided in the primary care setting, an area also explored in a large survey of diabetes care in general practice in England and Wales, published in July 2000. Further extensive work by the Audit Commission, relating to the delivery of services in primary and specialist diabetes care, has continued into 2001. Information and recommendations from the Report and current work will feed into the National Service Framework for Diabetes, due in 2001.

National Service Framework (NSF) for Diabetes

The NSF for Diabetes is expected to be published in 2001 with implementation commencing in April 2002. The Expert Reference Group presented its Advice to Ministers in April 2000, following extensive work and wide consultation. It is hoped that the NSF for Diabetes will include:

■ A new approach to the care of people with diabetes which encourages patient autonomy.

- Informed health care professionals working together to meet the needs of all those living with diabetes or caring for them.
- Identification and description of integrated care pathways in diabetes.
- Standards for diabetes care.
- Interventions that will achieve standards.
- A self-care model designed around the needs of the person with diabetes.
- A delivery strategy for implementation at national, regional, district, Primary Care Group/Trust and hospital trust levels.

References

Audit Commission (2000). *Testing Times: A review of diabetes services in England and Wales*. London: Audit Commission.

Cygnus Inc. (2001). *A Reference Manual for Health Professionals. Understanding the Glucowatch Automatic Biographer*. Redwood City (USA): Cygnus Inc.

Department of Health (2000). *The NHS Plan: A plan for investment, a plan for reform*. London: HMSO.

Diabetes UK (2001). *Annual Professional Conference Proceedings*. London: Diabetes UK.

Diabetes UK (2001). Annual Professional Meeting. Abstracts and Posters. *Diabetic Medicine* **18**: 2.

Owen OG (2001). Avenues of hope in the treatment of diabetes. *Hospital Doctor* 5 April: 46.

WHO (1998). *World Health*. Geneva: WHO.

Glossary

alpha cells	cells that produce glucagon in the islets of Langerhans in the pancreas
autonomic neuropathy	damage to the nervous system regulating the autonomic functions of the body
beef insulin	insulin extracted from the pancreas of cattle
beta cells (β cells)	cells that produce insulin in the islets of Langerhans in the pancreas
beta blockers	drugs that are used to treat angina and to lower blood pressure; they can change the warning signs of hypoglycaemia
biguanides	drugs used in treatment of diabetes; they lower blood glucose levels through increase in uptake of glucose by muscle, and reduction in absorption of glucose by the intestines and amount of glucose produced by liver
bovine insulin	insulin extracted from the pancreas of cattle
chiropodist	a practitioner of chiropody; also called a podiatrist
chiropody	specialty concerned with diagnosis and/or medical, surgical, mechanical, physical and adjunctive treatment of diseases, injuries and defects of the human foot; also called podiatry
DCCT	Diabetes Control and Complications Trial
diabetes insipidus	a disorder of the pituitary gland accompanied by excessive urination and thirst. These symptoms, although similar to those of diabetes mellitus, are **not** accompanied by hypoglycaemia
diabetes mellitus	a disorder of the pancreas characterised by high blood glucose levels, excessive urination and thirst, in addition to other signs and symptoms
diabetic amyotrophy	rare condition causing pain and/or weakness of the legs as a result of damage to certain nerves
diabetic coma	unconscious state characterised by severe hyperglycaemia, ketoacidosis and extreme biochemical imbalance
diabetic maculopathy	pathological disease of the eye caused by diabetes
diabetic nephropathy	renal damage caused by diabetes
diabetic neuropathy	nerve damage caused by diabetes
diabetic retinopathy	eye damage caused by diabetes
diuretics	agents that increase the flow of urine

exchanges	portions of carbohydrate foods that can be exchanged for one another. One exchange = 10 grams of carbohydrate
fructosamine	measurement of this indicates diabetes control, reflecting the average blood glucose level over the previous 2–3 weeks. Measurement of fructosamine should not be used to diagnose diabetes. *See* glycated haemoglobin
gestational diabetes	diabetes occurring during pregnancy but usually temporary
glaucoma	disease of the eye causing increased pressure inside the eye
glycosuria	presence of glucose in the urine
glycated haemoglobin (HbAlc)	this is the part of the haemoglobin that has glucose attached to it; measurement of HbA1c is a test of diabetes control, the amount depending on the average blood glucose level over the previous 2–3 months. Measurement of HbA1c should not be used to diagnose diabetes. *See* fructosamine
honeymoon period	occurring from weeks to months after the diagnosis of type 1 diabetes; less insulin is required during this period as a result of the partial recovery of insulin secretion by the pancreas
human insulin	insulin produced by recombinant technology which is close to and with a purity similar to the human species
hyperglycaemia	high blood glucose level: >12 mmol/l
hypo	abbreviation for hypoglycaemia
hypoglycaemia	low blood glucose level: < 3.5 mmol/l
Hypostop gel	glucose/dextrose gel that can be rubbed on gums of diabetic person undergoing a hypoglycaemic episode, and is particularly useful if the patient is uncooperative; available on prescription (FP10)
incidence	the number of new cases of a disease occurring during a given time period, usually expressed as new cases per 100,000 of the population per year
IDDM	insulin-dependent diabetes mellitus – *see* type 1 diabetes
IFG	impaired fasting glycaemia
IGT	impaired glucose tolerance
impaired fasting glycaemia	this is a new category, which includes people with fasting glucose levels above normal, but not enough to diagnose diabetes, i.e. between 6.1 and 7.0 mmol/l
impaired glucose tolerance	indicated by a fasting venous glucose value of 6–8 mmol/l. Confirmed by an OGGT of >7.8 mmol/l, but <11.1 mmol/l or a fasting plasma glucose of <7.0 mmol/l
insulin coma	severe hypoglycaemia causing the unconscious state and sometimes convulsions
insulin pen	device that resembles a large fountain pen that takes a cartridge of insulin. Injection of insulin occurs after dialling the dose and pressing a button

intermediate-acting insulin	insulin preparation with action lasting 12–18 hours
islets of Langerhans	specialised cells within the pancreas that produce insulin and glucagon
isophane	a form of intermediate-acting insulin that has protamine added to slow its absorption
juvenile-onset diabetes	outdated name for type 1 diabetes. Most patients who receive insulin develop it before the age of 40. This term is no longer in use
ketoacidosis	a serious condition resulting from lack of insulin which, in turn, results in body fat being used to produce energy, forming ketones and acids; it is characterised by high blood glucose levels, ketones in the urine, vomiting, drowsiness, heavy laboured breathing and a smell of acetone on the breath
ketonuria	presence of acetone and other ketones in the urine; detected by testing with Ketostix. Occurs in association with severe hyperglycaemia or in the starving state
lente insulin	a form of intermediate-acting insulin that has zinc added to slow its absorption
lipoatrophy	loss of fat from injection sites; used to occur before use of highly purified insulins
lipohypertrophy	fatty swelling usually caused by repeated injections of insulin into the same site
maculopathy	pathological disease of the eye
maturity-onset diabetes	outdated term for type 2 diabetes, most commonly occurring in people who are middle-aged and overweight
metabolic syndrome	a cluster of medical problems – diabetes, hypertension, central obesity, abnormal lipids, coronary heart disease
microalbuminuria	excretion of minute traces of protein in the urine, in amounts undetectable using dipsticks; an indicator of early, possibly treatable, renal disease
nephropathy	kidney damage; initially this causes the kidney to 'leak' so that albumin appears in the urine. Later it may affect kidney function and in severe cases lead to kidney failure
neuropathy	damage to the nerves, which may be peripheral or autonomic neuropathy
NIDDM	non-insulin-dependent diabetes mellitus – *see* type 2 diabetes
oral glucose tolerance test (OGTT)	test used in the diagnosis of diabetes mellitus; glucose in the blood is measured at intervals before and after the person has drunk a measured amount of glucose after a high-carbohydrate load and fasting before the test. Also used to screen for IGT
PCDUK	Primary Care Diabetes UK (see Appendix IV)

peripheral neuropathy	damage to the nerves supplying the muscles and skin; can result in diminished sensation and vibration perception, particularly feet and legs. Muscle weakness may also follow
podiatrist	*see* chiropodist
podiatry	*see* chiropody
polyuria	passing of large quantities of urine as a result of excess glucose in the bloodstream; a symptom of untreated diabetes mellitus (and diabetes insipidus)
porcine insulin	insulin extracted from the pancreas of pigs
PPGRs	postprandial glucose regulators, e.g. repaglinide: drugs that reduce blood glucose levels. They have a similar mode of action to sulphonylureas, but with a faster onset and shorter duration of action
prevalence	the number of cases of a disease at a given point in time, expressed as a proportion of the population
proteinuria	protein or albumin in the urine
RCGP	Royal College of General Practitioners
RCP	Royal College of Physicians
renal threshold	the level of glucose in the blood above which it will start to spill into the urine, causing glycosuria; the threshold in normal subjects is 10 mmol/l (blood glucose level). In all subjects, the renal threshold rises with age
retinopathy	damage to the retina
rosiglitazone	one of the thiazolidinediones
short-acting insulin	insulin preparations with action lasting 6–12 hours
Snellen chart	chart used to assess visual acuity
sulphonylureas	drugs that lower the blood glucose levels by stimulating the pancreatic β cells to produce more insulin, e.g. tolbutamide, gliclazide
thiazolidinediones	drugs (also called PPAR-gamma agonists and glitazones) that reduce blood glucose and insulin levels. This is achieved by a reduction in insulin resistance, resulting in increased effectiveness of available insulin in liver, fat and muscle
type 1 diabetes	type of diabetes that must be treated with insulin; also known as insulin-dependent diabetes mellitus (IDDM)
type 2 diabetes	type of diabetes that occurs in older people (>40 years), particularly if overweight; these people do not always need insulin treatment and can usually be controlled successfully with diet alone or diet and drugs; also called non-insulin-dependent diabetes mellitus (NIDDM). When treated with insulin, the term used is insulin-treated type 2 diabetes
UKPDS	UK Prospective Diabetes Study

Part I

Diabetes: an overview

Responsibilities of those involved in the provision of diabetes care

■ The role of the practice nurse in general practice diabetes care
■ The evolving role of the practice nurse in integrated diabetes care
■ The role of other members of the health care team in primary diabetes care
■ The role of receptionists, clerical staff and practice managers

The general practitioner

The general practitioner takes overall clinical responsibility for the provision of care. In addition, the GP, as an employer, is bound by the code of conduct of the General Medical Council. In employing practice nurses, the doctors 'must be satisfied that the person to whom they delegate duties is competent to carry out such treatments and procedures'.

In diabetes care, the GP's involvement will, to some extent, depend on his or her interest in and commitment to the subject. Responsibility for the practice diabetes service may be carried by the doctor or shared/integrated.

To obtain Band 3 level reimbursement, the GP is required to incorporate the national guidance on health promotion/chronic disease management guidelines introduced in July 1993. These guidelines are more flexible than the previous scheme, allowing practices more freedom in designing programmes to suit the particular needs of their patients.

The GP's role and responsibilities in diabetes care include:

■ Providing appropriate medical services.
■ Ensuring that a full medical review and laboratory/other tests are carried out after diagnosis.
■ Instituting an initial programme of treatment, support, education and surveillance after diagnosis, and at annual review, with the practice and community nurse and others, as appropriate.
■ Abiding by locally agreed criteria for referral, ensuring that referrals to specialist teams or other agencies are timely and appropriate.
■ In association with other members of the primary care team, ensuring that good communication exists between all parties involved, verbally and in writing.

- Ensuring that other medical problems are taken into account in relation to diabetes management.
- Together with the practice nurse, community nurse and members of the team, enabling people with diabetes (and their families and carers) to be informed and supported sufficiently to empower them to control their own diabetes health and to lead as healthy a life as possible.

The practice nurse

The practice nurse (or community nurse, if involved) is professionally account-able for any nursing service provided, as laid down by the UKCC. In a specialist subject, such as diabetes, where particular knowledge (further to that gained in pre-registration training and/or acquired only in hospital care or outside a general practice setting) is necessary, it is important that items 3 and 4 in the UKCC Code of Professional Conduct are given particular consideration.

No. 3: 'Maintain and improve your professional knowledge and competence.'

No. 4: 'Acknowledge any limitations in your knowledge and competence and decline any duties or responsibilities unless able to perform them in a safe and skilled manner.'

Further information
UKCC, 23 Portland Place, London W1N 3AF
Telephone: 020 7637 7181

Indemnity for practice nurses

For practice nurses who have not taken up any indemnity, this is offered by the Royal College of Nursing or the Medical Defence Union.

The role of the practice nurse in general practice diabetes care

Nurses have been employed in general practice since 1911, but not in any num-ber until the late 1960s after a large financial input to general practice which allowed expansion of care. In 1978 there were 3,100 and in 1984 over 6,000 nurses employed part- or whole-time in general practice. This figure has increased to over 18,000 since 1990 with changes in the National Health Service.

The role of the practice nurse has undoubtedly changed and extended with the expansion of developments in the promotion of health and the prevention and management of disease. The role encompasses four important elements in the care of the local population (Fig. 1.1):

1. Personal contact
2. Care provision
3. Coordinating function
4. Flexibility.

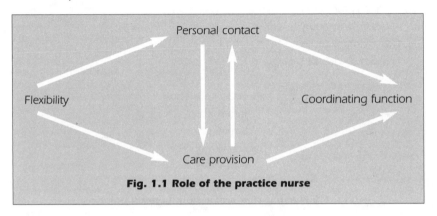

Fig. 1.1 Role of the practice nurse

Personal contact

Easy and regular contact with patients is important in preventive care. Fostering good relationships with families, businesses and local services, and building 'networks' takes time and entails hard work. Rewards are, however, there when a patient benefits from the results, perhaps by meeting another with a similar problem or by being put in touch with an organisation or self-help group.

Within a practice, the nurse may at times be the only health care professional on the premises when doctors are out on visits. In a large practice with many doctors and staff employed, contact with the nurse may be easier, particularly during busy surgeries or where the patient is concerned about 'bothering' the doctor.

Care provision

The nursing service provided in general practice allows all aspects of care of the individual and the family to be encompassed (Fig. 1.2). These involve many activities linked by the four elements of listening, supporting, advising and teaching/explaining.

The organisation of such a workload is an important aspect of practice nursing particularly in keeping track of patients – and providing the necessary follow-up care after an attendance or telephone call requesting help.

First aid/emergencies
Accident prevention
Immunisation
Children
Travel

Health promotion	LISTEN	Treatment/procedures
Health education		Screening
Disease management	SUPPORT	Medicals
Health surveillance	ADVISE	Investigations
		Counselling

Information collection
Information
dissemination
Liaison with outside
agencies

Fig. 1.2 Nursing care provided in general practice.

Coordinating function

The practice nurse has an important role within the practice in the education of other members of the practice team with regard to raising awareness of problems, the tracking of patients, fostering good working relationships and communicating with other team members. It is in these areas in general practice that difficulties sometimes arise, preventing the effective delivery of health care (Fig. 1.3).

The nurse's role in coordinating care and services 'outside' the practice is also important, particularly in relation to diabetes, where many other health care professionals and supporting services may be required in the provision of care over a person's lifetime with the condition.

Flexibility

Of all conditions, diabetes requires a flexible system of care from diagnosis. As far as possible, independence, choice and flexibility are 'key' factors in support, education and surveillance. In general practice, the nurse is the 'key' person to provide these elements.

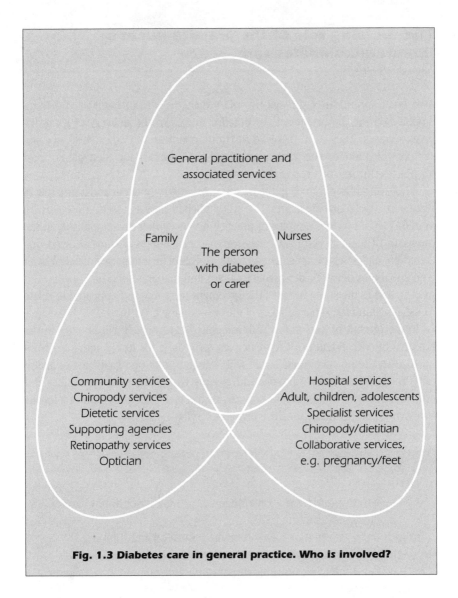

General practitioner and
associated services

Family

The person
with diabetes
or carer

Nurses

Community services
Chiropody services
Dietetic services
Supporting agencies
Retinopathy services
Optician

Hospital services
Adult, children, adolescents
Specialist services
Chiropody/dietitian
Collaborative services,
e.g. pregnancy/feet

Fig. 1.3 Diabetes care in general practice. Who is involved?

Another example of flexibility encompassed by practice nurses is the group of people with diabetes who attend neither hospital nor general practice except when they are 'ill'. This may be because they are elderly, disabled or unaware that they require health care for their diabetes. This group may not be visited by any health care professional except in an emergency situation. The practice nurse, having identified the group, can take 'diabetes care' to the patient's home, arrange appropriate investigations, check that 'all is well' in the house, and if not arrange appropriate support and a follow-up visit from the general practitioner at least annually.

The evolving role of the practice nurse in integrated diabetes care

A national enquiry in a survey of primary diabetes care in England and Wales emphasised the important role of practice nurses in the delivery of local diabetes services. They were involved in running almost all dedicated clinics and ran one-third alone. The study highlighted the necessity for adequate support for practice nurses involved in diabetes care.

A two-round Delphi study in the UK enquired into the current and future role of nurses in type 2 diabetes care. The study elicited and assessed consensus on opinions from random samples of practice nurses with a substantial role in the provision of diabetes care and diabetes specialist nurses. Results showed that there were high levels of agreement on many aspects of the future care of people with type 2 diabetes between the practice nurses and diabetes specialist nurses who participated in the study. Areas of disagreement were few and appeared to relate to issues around the separate roles of the two nursing groups.

In the pursuit of person-centred, integrated care, which will be core to the National Service Framework for Diabetes, proposed for implementation from April 2002, the practice nurse's role will change to that of a facilitator of health care. The practice nurse will work with people with diabetes, their families and other care providers, and across boundaries to ensure the provision of a locally supportive and culturally sensitive diabetes service.

SUMMARY

- The practice nurse has a key role in the provision of primary care diabetes services in the UK.
- It is important that practice nurses are educated and supported.
- His or her relationship and knowledge of the person with diabetes and family members enables contact with general practitioners and other providers of care.
- Relationships and trust are built which encourage clinic attendance.
- The practice nurse is in an ideal position to organise and coordinate a protected but flexible service in the practice setting.
- In the delivery of person-centred, integrated diabetes care in the future, the role of the practice nurse will expand and evolve, in line with the development of other roles for nurses as described in the Department of Health NHS Plan.

The role of other members of the health care team in primary diabetes care

The community (district) nurse

The community nurse may have a similar role to the practice nurse, although providing diabetes care at home. Clinical provision by community nurses may involve any of the following:

- General assessment of health care needs.
- Overall monitoring and surveillance – especially for frail, elderly people living alone.
- Administration or supervision of the administration of insulin at home.
- Support for and education of those newly diagnosed, treated with insulin and/or those caring for them.
- Providing or supervising care for those disabled by complications of diabetes.
- Treating/dressing diabetic foot ulcers.
- Monitoring blood glucose control as necessary.
- Liaising with the practice and/or specialist team regarding specific problems and the overall care of the person concerned.

The dietitian

The role of the dietitian is discussed in Chapter 7.

The chiropodist (podiatrist)

The role of the chiropodist is discussed in Chapter 11.

The counsellor and psychotherapist

Psychological support may be required at a level that cannot be provided by the GP or primary care nurses. It is important that the need for psychological health care is recognised and that referrals are sensitively handled.

The community psychiatric team

It is recognised that there may be an intercurrent psychiatric illness (clinical depression) coexisting with a life-long medical condition that is progressive, as in diabetes mellitus. The services provided by the community psychiatric team may be helpful in the supervision of the treatment in the home setting.

The optician (optometrist)

The role of the optician is discussed in Chapter 10.

The community pharmacist

Community pharmacists are increasingly involved in community health care. Regarding diabetes care, they may:

■ Offer advice after consultation
■ Dispense prescriptions
■ Provide supplies (insulin pens/needles, blood glucose monitors/equipment and foot care products) for sale
■ Operate a service for disposal of sharps
■ Provide facilities for customers to weigh themselves
■ Liaise with other community pharmacists, the primary care team and secondary care services
■ Deliver prescriptions to the home
■ Provide out-of-hours/emergency pharmacy services
■ Advise on drugs including doses, timing, administration routes, side effects, interactions and disposal.

The community link worker

Health care for specific ethnic populations, who may have language, culture and other personal barriers to overcome, will be improved where suitably trained link workers are included in the team and are available when needed.

Note: not all members of the primary care team who might be involved in providing care are necessarily included here. It is also important to recognise that members of the diabetes team may be involved in primary diabetes care, bridging the gap between primary and specialist services, e.g. diabetes specialist nurses, facilitators, 'specialist' dietitians and chiropodists (podiatrists).

The role of receptionists, clerical staff and practice managers

Administrative staff in a practice have increasing responsibilities. Most important are those in contact every day with patients, relatives and visitors to the practice, either in person or by telephone.

Receptionists are definitely 'front line'. Their attitude, knowledge and understanding of the problems of people telephoning or attending the practice may have a bearing on whether help is sought when needed.

Clerical staff also have an important part to play in the secretarial and administrative aspects of health care – particularly where computerisation of prescriptions, information, registers and recall systems has been implemented.

In small practices, there may only be a small administrative workforce who know the small practice population well and can very quickly identify those with diabetes. In a large practice or a practice with several branch surgeries, there may be many part-time staff working in shifts with communications passed from one to the other in writing. It is unlikely in this situation that the 'front line' will have as much knowledge of their diabetic population.

Larger practices have for many years required the employment of a practice manager to run the business side of the practice. Fund-holding practices, whether singularly or in groups, are looking at provision of care and costs associated with their practices, as well as an expanding workforce. The practice manager has an increasing responsibility in these developments.

An understanding of the roles and responsibilities of administrative staff is important in diabetes care in general practice. Education of the practice manager, receptionists and clerical staff about diabetes, the treatment and acute problems requiring immediate access to the doctor or nurse enables an understanding of the problems encountered by people with diabetes and dispels some of the fear, ignorance, mystery and 'old wives' tales' surrounding this condition.

Administrative staff are in a unique position in the identification of the diabetic population with their knowledge of those attending the practice, as receivers of information and in the organisation of prescriptions. Accurate input of information regarding demography, care provision, treatment changes and other data to computer systems is vital in the audit of diabetes care and in the assessment of needs for the future.

Further reading

Audit Commission (2000). *Testing Times: A review of diabetes services in England and Wales*. London: Audit Commission.

Department of Health (2000). *The NHS Plan: A plan for investment, a plan for reform.* London: HMSO.

MacKinnon M (2001–2002). The role of the practice nurse in diabetes care. *RCGP Members' Reference Book.* London: Campden Publishing Ltd.

Peters J, Hutchinson A, MacKinnon M, McIntosh A, Cooke J, Jones R (2001). What role do nurses play in Type 2 diabetes care in the community: a Delphi study. *Journal of Advanced Nursing* 34: 179–88

Pierce M, Agarwal G, Ridout D (2000). A survey of diabetes care in general practice in England and Wales. *British Journal of General Practice* 50: 542–5

2 Educational needs of the team

- Diabetes education for the primary care team – what is available?
- Diabetes education for the primary health care team – what is needed?

In a complex subject such as diabetes, an up-to-date knowledge and the appropriate application of knowledge are necessary for the clinical management and education of people with diabetes. Often doctors and nurses are not aware of their own continuing educational needs in order to provide the support and correct, consistent information essential for people managing their own care.

In order to ascertain educational requirements of those involved (mainly doctors and nurses), it may be helpful for members of the 'team' to identify their own learning needs by checking a 'diabetes topic' list (Fig. 2.1). This list is not inclusive of every topic, but encompasses many subjects, where clinical management, information and explanation are reliant on a level of knowledge which might be expected of the doctor or nurse, by a person with diabetes, newly diagnosed or during their diabetic life. It is understood that it is sometimes difficult to know what 'you don't know'. The list is aimed to stimulate enquiry.

Fig. 2.1 Diabetes knowledge – needs assessment

Please fill in the appropriate space using the following key:

0 = No knowledge of topic
1 = Some knowledge of topic – Insufficient
2 = Good knowledge of topic – Sufficient

_____	Types of diabetes	_____	Hypos
_____	Causes of diabetes	_____	Practical aspects
_____	Inheritance	_____	Unproven methods of
		_____	treatment
_____	Physiology	_____	Alternative therapy
_____	Symptoms	_____	Control

Fig. 2.1 contd

_____ Related conditions	_____ Monitoring
_____ Diet	_____ Blood glucose
_____ Overweight	_____ Urine glucose
_____ Tablets	_____ Glycated Hb
_____ Insulin	_____ Thrush
_____ Management (of diabetes care)	_____ HRT
_____ Brittle diabetes	_____ Termination of pregnancy
_____ Sport	_____ Infertility
_____ Eating out	_____ Genetics
_____ Holidays	_____ Pre-pregnancy
_____ Travel	_____ Pregnancy
_____ Work	_____ Gestational diabetes
_____ Other illness	_____ Baby with diabetes
_____ Sick day rules	_____ Child with diabetes
_____ Surgical operations	_____ Diabetes in adolescence
_____ Investigations	_____ A cure?
_____ Driving	_____ Complications
_____ Alcohol	_____ Feet, footwear
_____ Drugs	_____ Chiropody
_____ Smoking	_____ Retinopathy
_____ Impotence	_____ Vision
_____ Contraception	_____ Transplantation
_____ Hypertension	_____ Insulin pumps
_____ Cardiovascular problems	_____ Artificial pancreas
_____ Psychological aspects	_____ New insulins
_____ Diabetes UK	_____ Oral insulins
Emergency treatment _____ of hyperglycaemia	Emergencies
_____ Life insurance	Emergency treatment _____ of hypoglycaemia
_____ Fructosamine	_____ Medical insurance

Members of the team may find it helpful to score themselves and note further topics of identified educational need.

_____

_____

_____

_____

_____

_____

_____

Diabetes education for the primary care team – what is available?

The St Vincent Joint Task Force Subgroup Report on Training and Professional Development in Diabetes Care (1996) recognises the many professions providing diabetes care, and the diversity and levels involved in their professional training and continuing education. Particular skills are required to provide the clinical, educational and psychological care of people with diabetes and their families.

Following the St Vincent Report, Diabetes UK has set up a Professional Development Project. This will become a resource and a framework for all professionals providing diabetes care, enabling them to learn and use the necessary skills identified in the Report.

Diabetes courses

Integrated or planned courses

These are usually based in a centre with a well-developed clinical base and diabetes nurse specialist involvement:

- Length
  - half-day workshops
  - study days
  - 2–3 days
  - weekends
  - evenings over several weeks
- Evaluation – brief to detailed questionnaires
- Style and content – variable, some didactic, academic and hospital based.

One-off events

These are usually organised by a diabetes nurse specialist using 'soft' money.

Courses in academic institutions

English National Board Course No. 928 in Diabetic Nursing: details from the English National Board for Nursing, Midwifery and Health Visiting (see page 297).

Modules on diabetes: incorporated into other nursing courses: these are validated and may lead to a practice nurse attendance certificate/diploma or community nurse qualification/diploma.

Institutions offering courses:

- Colleges of nursing
- Colleges of health
- Institutes of health
- Colleges of further education
- Universities.

Distance learning courses

It has been recognised that there are problems for health care professionals taking time away from their clinical service, particularly those working in the primary health care setting. Training budgets are tight. The mandatory training requirements for nurses for PREP (UKCC) are a total of 5 days over 3 years. For practice and continuity nurses, distance learning courses are popular. They may include other members of the primary care team and should have appropriate educational accreditation. Apply to Diabetes UK for details of distance learning and other accredited courses.

Professional educational requirements

For nurses

- There are many developing diploma, degree and higher degree courses – in which diabetes may be a part or module.
- Credits or CAT points should be available on all validated courses where assessment is integral to the course.
- PREP and ENB Higher Award Schemes should make continuing education more available for all nurses.
- District diabetes care should include, in any strategy, the recognition of the need for local training and continuing education for nurses in primary care teams.
- Local or district schemes should be planned by specialist teams in conjunction with academic/continuing education institutions.

Short courses

Diabetic Course for Community Nurses
Department of Nursing and Midwifery, University of Glasgow, 68 Oakfield Avenue, Glasgow G12 8LS
Run twice a year. Contact Ms Joan McDowell, tel: 0141 339 8855

ENB 928 Short Course in Diabetic Nursing for Nurses, Midwives and Health Visitors on all Parts of the Professional Register
English National Board for Nursing, Midwifery and Health Visiting, London
Courses run throughout the year; contact: NHS Careers, PO Box 376, Bristol BS99 3EY, tel: 0845 606 0655.

ENB AO5 The Care of Patients with Diabetes
10-day course run over a year.

ENB N97 Diabetes Nursing in Primary Health Care Settings
Course run over 25 days.

Multidisciplinary (certificate and diploma courses) (part distance learning)

Certificate in Diabetes Care
University of Warwick, Coventry CV4 7AL
Contact: Rachel Winnington, tel: 024 7657 2958

Diabetes Management in Primary Care (Diploma)
DTC Primary Care Training Centre, Shipley, W. Yorkshire
Run every 2 months; contact: Sarah Maylor, tel: 01274 617617

Working with Physical Illness: a systemic approach
Tavistock Clinic, London. Contact: Academic Services, tel: 020 7447 3718

Working with Families and Teams – an introduction to systems-based approaches in general practice
Tavistock Clinic, London. Contact: Academic Services, tel: 020 7447 3718

Masters courses over a longer period

MA/MSc Applied Health Studies (Diabetes care)
University of Warwick, Coventry
A new (2001) flexible masters programme that addresses the higher educational needs of health care professionals involved in the delivery of integrated diabetes care. The programme supports the achievement of the standards of care identified in the National Service Framework for Diabetes in the UK, as well as the educational needs of health care professionals at an international level.
For information, contact Warwick Diabetes Care, tel: 024 7657 2958

Masters in Clinical Science (Diabetes)
University of Warwick, Coventry
Modular diabetes diploma and masters courses (with modules as stand-alone postgraduate awards) for health care professionals. These courses became available in October 2001. For information contact Warwick Diabetes Care, tel: 024 7657 2958

Postgraduate Diploma in Diabetes Care for Healthcare Professionals
University of Exeter
Module programme of two taught and one self-directed learning modules (one day per week). Run over one year; contact: Institute of General Practice, University of Exeter

Graduate Certificated/Graduate Diploma/Masters in Diabetes
Chelsea & Westminster Hospital, 369 Fulham Road, London/University of Surrey, Roehampton
Run once a year, also run a distance learning course; tel: 020 8237 2731 or 020 8392 3562

Self-help for the primary care team

- Organise own education by attending courses/conferences.
- Find a 'buddy' practice to befriend and learn and share experiences.
- Locate a 'mentor' practice with long experience of provision of diabetes care.
- Contact the local diabetes team and request resources and education.
- Contact Diabetes UK for further information.
- Driving and diabetes: see the Diabetes UK leaflet.
- Join Diabetes UK.

Mainly for general practitioners

- Postgraduate course in diabetes held annually – changing centres every 2–3 years. Details from specialist diabetes physicians or Diabetes UK.
- Local initiatives – through General Practitioner Training Schemes, Postgraduate Centres, RCGP Training, Diabetes Team Initiatives (PGEA schemes usually sought).
- Warwick Diabetes Care (University of Warwick) – a coherent point of contact for all those involved in providing diabetes care in the following ways: providing and promoting multidisciplinary diabetes education courses for health care professionals; undertaking and supporting applied diabetes research; developing practical resources and people networks.

SUMMARY

1. Diabetes education for the primary health care team is available in some areas. Availability, accessibility and educational level are, however, variable and often reliant on 'soft' money.

2. The messages from general practice are that education is best when practice based and related to the work and development of each primary health care team. There is thus a major need for co-ordination in each district among the consumers (PHCTs), the diabetes provider teams and the education institutions, and a willingness on the part of 'specialists' in diabetes to tailor their knowledge appropriately to the local community, where this is needed. Training and continuing education should be reflected in local contracting arrangements.

Diabetes education for the primary health care team – what is needed?

The following units provide the basis for a primary care team course allowing participants to develop their knowledge and practice of diabetes care. Practical skills and the techniques used in motivational interviewing (see Chapter 13) are also required.

Unit 1: diabetes mellitus – an overview of the condition

Aim

To provide an opportunity for the team to obtain an overview of diabetes including the progress and treatment of the condition.

Objectives

1. Examine the physiology, aetiology and clinical picture of diabetes.
2. Discuss the epidemiology of diabetes.
3. Consider current research into diabetes and its implications in the delivery of future care.
4. Consider the available approaches for the control of blood glucose and prevention of extremes of blood glucose levels.
5. In the practice context, explore methods of screening, diagnosis and criteria for referral.

6. Examine the three modes of treatment (the food plan, medication and insulin) and their delivery in the context of age and lifestyle.
7. Identify problems of management of the control of weight, blood glucose levels and blood pressure in the ongoing care of the person with diabetes.
8. Specify the difficulties encountered by the newly diagnosed (and the family/carers) in terms of management, education and support.
9. Construct a practice guideline for the management of intercurrent illness in the person with diabetes.
10. Consider the complications of diabetes, surveillance and identification of those at risk including treatment and criteria for referral.

Unit 2: living with diabetes

Aim

To enable the team to explore and understand the psychological and social implications of living with diabetes.

Objectives

1. Gain greater insight into the implications of diabetes for the lifestyle of people with diabetes and their families/carers by listening to them.
2. Develop an understanding of the problems and management in different age groups and during pregnancy.
3. Recognise the need for support and the resources available to meet this need.
4. Examine critically the role of education in diabetes care.
5. Consider the organisation and function of the hospital services, the general practice services and diabetes centres in the delivery of care.
6. Identify the role of other health care professionals in diabetes care and the pathways of referral to them.
7. Explore the important role of voluntary organisations in diabetes care, in particular the role of Diabetes UK.

Unit 3: the management of diabetes care in general practice

Aim

To provide an opportunity for the primary health care team to examine their own practice management of diabetes care.

Objectives

1. Identify the aims and objectives of the practice diabetes service.
2. Discuss the purpose of the diabetes service in general practice.
3. Specify the skills required to run the service.
4. Analyse the organisation required.
5. Describe methods of evaluation and audit of the service.
6. Consider the identification and systems for registration, follow-up and recall of people with diabetes in the practice.
7. Design realistic and effective educational aims and objectives applicable to the practice diabetes population.
8. Construct protocols for:
   (a) initial assessment of newly diagnosed patients
   (b) a routine review
   (c) an annual review.
9. List short- and long-term aims for the practice diabetes service.
10. Explore methods of 'team work' in terms of working together and problem solving.

Further reading

British Diabetic Association (1997). *Recommendations for Management of Diabetes in Primary Care*. London: BDA.

British Diabetic Association Specialist UK Working Group Reports (1996). St Vincent and improving diabetes care. *Diabetic Medicine* **13** (9) (suppl 4): 65–76.

Roberts S, MacKinnon M, Braid E (1992). Draft report on educational initiatives in diabetes for general practitioners and their teams. Unpublished report. London: British Diabetic Association, Education Section.

Diabetes mellitus in the United Kingdom

■ Prevalence and incidence
■ The consequences of diabetes
■ Mortality
■ The cost of diabetes
■ The aims of diabetes care
■ Diabetes UK

Prevalence and incidence

The prevalence of diabetes in the United Kingdom suggested by most authorities is 3% or more. Undiagnosed diabetes existing in the population may account for a further 2%. The prevalence of diabetes is considerably increased in certain ethnic groups (south Asians, i.e. Asians from the Indian subcontinent, and African–Caribbeans) and is higher in the older age range of all ethnic groups. Over the age of 75 years, this figure may increase to as much as 10% of the population. The increase in prevalence of diabetes in the UK population relating to age is shown in Fig. 3.1.

Figures available for the prevalence of diabetes in children and young people (under the age of 11 years) show that this condition has become more common over the last 20 years and that the increase is mainly in social classes I and II. The prevalence of type 1 diabetes (insulin-dependent diabetes) in people under the age of 20 years is 0.14% (1.4 per 1,000) which means that there are probably more than 20,000 young people with diabetes in the United Kingdom. There is a rising trend for incidence of diabetes in this age group.

People with type 2 diabetes (non-insulin-dependent diabetes) may remain undiagnosed for months or years. The condition may be diagnosed only by coincidence, after routine screening (e.g. at a medical examination, a routine outpatient visit or before surgery).

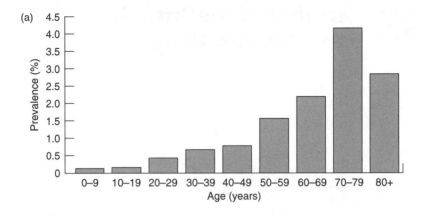

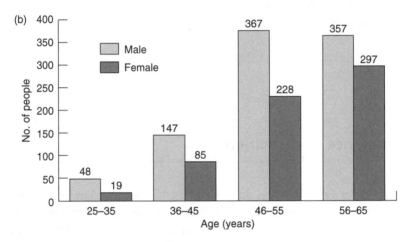

Fig. 3.1 (a) The age-specific prevalence of diagnosed diabetes in the Oxford Community Study. (b) The age and sex distribution of people entering the UK Prospective Diabetes Study

The number of new cases of diabetes diagnosed each year in the UK is estimated to be 60,000 (Diabetes UK). In the UK there are about 1,380,000 adults with known diabetes; most of these have type 2 diabetes mellitus (75–90%). It is estimated that there are 1 million people with diabetes undiagnosed in the UK (Diabetes UK Report 'Missing Million').

Racial variations

High rates of diabetes are found in the south Asian population in the UK (those Asians originating from the Indian subcontinent). The prevalence is approximately four times higher than that found in the white population. The prevalence of diabetes in south Asians is further increased with age, to as much as 16% in the 40–65 age range – four to five times higher than the white population of similar age.

African–Caribbean people in the UK also have a slightly higher prevalence of type 2 diabetes, associated with weight gain.

Both these populations are more at risk of cardiac disease, a significant complication of diabetes.

The consequences of diabetes

Retinopathy

Surveys show that 30% of all people with diabetes have retinopathy and about 1–2% develop sight-threatening changes each year; the prevalence rises to about 80% after 20 years of diabetes. If these are detected early enough, usually before vision is affected, laser treatment will prevent 70% from going blind. In 1980, diabetes was the most common cause of blindness in people aged 45–64 years. People with diabetes in that age group were 23 times more likely to be blind than their non-diabetic contemporaries. Over 65 years, they are twice as likely to be blind.

Nephropathy

Diabetic nephropathy is a major cause of morbidity and mortality in patients with type 1 diabetes mellitus, and affects some 40% of patients who develop diabetes before they are 30 years old. The cumulative mortality after 30 years of diabetes is about 12%. A survey in 1985 found that 580 people with diabetes in the UK developed renal failure. About 450 were thought suitable for treatment, but it was only possible to provide dialysis or transplantation for about 270 of them.

Neuropathy

Evidence of neuropathy may be found in up to 40% of people with diabetes (30% of those in hospital studies but over 50% of patients with type 2 diabetes), causing problems for about one-third of them. One of the most distressing and often hidden problems is that of male impotence, which can affect one in two men with diabetes by varying degrees of erectile dysfunction.

Foot ulceration

Foot ulceration is at least 50 times more common in people with diabetes than in the non-diabetic population. If the ulceration is the result of peripheral vascular disease, amputation is often the outcome. Over the age of 65 years, people with diabetes are 25 times more likely to have had a leg amputated than those without diabetes. Collaborative foot clinics have shown that with a specialist team approach the need for amputation can be halved.

Mortality

It is recognised that people with diabetes die earlier than those of a similar age and sex without the condition. Death may be directly caused by diabetes (e.g. diabetic ketoacidosis or renal failure resulting from diabetes). More commonly, however, death is caused by macrovascular complications, particularly myocardial infarctions and strokes.

It is suggested that about 40,000 people with diabetes die each year in the UK. If analysed by age and sex, it seems that about 20,000 die prematurely each year as the result of having diabetes. Premature deaths are more marked in women than in men and more obvious in the younger age groups. The number of people with diabetes dying prematurely is twice that of the non-diabetic population. Deaths occur as a result of one of the causes in the box below.

- Cardiovascular disease
- Strokes
- Kidney failure
- Peripheral vascular disease
- Diabetic ketoacidosis

A study of death in 448 people with diabetes under the age of 50 years from various parts of the UK was carried out in 1979. In this survey, the two most common causes of death of people with diabetes under the age of 50 were heart attacks and kidney failure. In those aged under 20 years, ketoacidosis is the most common cause of death.

Cardiovascular disease

Overall, people with diabetes are more likely to die of heart attacks than people without diabetes. In men there is a two- to threefold increased risk of coronary heart disease than in non-diabetic people; in premenopausal women the risk is four- to fivefold. In younger patients (under 45) the increased risk of dying from a heart attack is much greater, five times more likely in men and 11.5 times more likely in women. Nephropathy is a significant risk factor.

Strokes

Women with diabetes are twice as likely to die from strokes, men about 1.5 times more likely. There is an increased risk of mortality from strokes in younger people with diabetes.

Kidney failure

This is a common cause of death in those who develop diabetes before they are 30 years old. In a survey of people dying from kidney failure before 50 years of age, death was found to be 40 times more common in people with diabetes. Recent surveys have, however, shown that, as treatment has improved over the last 40 years, the incidence of nephropathy and kidney failure has decreased by about one-third. Renal failure can now be treated by dialysis or renal transplantation.

Peripheral vascular disease

Although the number of deaths among people with diabetes from this cause is not so high, there are about 2.5 times more deaths than would be expected in non-diabetic individuals of the same age and sex.

Diabetic ketoacidosis

In the 1979 survey carried out by the then British Diabetic Association and the Royal College of Physicians, 74 of the 448 people with diabetes studied died from diabetic ketoacidosis. If this condition does develop, early treatment should lead to the condition being corrected. Death in these patients was often the result of psychological problems and delays in treatment. Ketoacidosis was the most common cause of death in people with diabetes aged under 20. The most common causes of severe ketoacidosis remain delay in diagnosing type 1 diabetes and misplaced advice given sometimes to people to stop their insulin during intercurrent illness, when they are vomiting or not eating.

The cost of diabetes

In the UK, in 1989, people with diabetes consumed between 4% and 5% of health care resources. The cost of diabetes to the NHS was estimated to have been £1 billion. Patients with diabetes have a hospital bed occupancy of about double that for all other categories of patients combined. This excludes community nursing services or primary care where diabetes is not the primary diagnosis.

The King's Fund report on the impact and costs of diabetes showed in 1997 that 10% of all health care costs will be spent on diabetes care in the future, and that this will inevitably go up with the projected increases in numbers of people developing diabetes. Direct costs to the NHS include inpatient and outpatient care provided by hospitals, services provided by general practitioners and district nurses in the community, and the cost of supplies – insulin, tablets, syringes, needle clippers and monitoring strips. In addition, there are costs involved, particularly in screening for and treating retinopathy, in the treatment of end-stage renal failure and the special costs incurred by those who have suffered amputation.

Indirect costs to the individual of unfulfilled ambitions, the psychological effect of combined anxieties about living with diabetes and the prospect of developing complications cannot be quantified. The costs of loss of earning capacity resulting from ill health or premature death are unknown, although estimated to be significant compared with the non-diabetic population.

Good evidence is available that regional costs could be reduced by a number of inexpensive measures. For example:

1. The provision of sufficient interested and trained physicians and nurses working with dietitians and chiropodists/podiatrists.
2. Adequate education facilities for people with diabetes and their families.
3. Resources and support for general practitioners and their teams caring for the non-hospital diabetic population.

Reducing the costs of diabetes may be achieved through:

- Primary prevention
- Prevention of complications
- Implementation of agreed standards of care
- Reduction in inappropriate admissions to hospital
- Examination of the costs and benefits of the management, screening and treatment options available.

Effectiveness of treatment for people with diabetes

The maintenance of near physiological blood glucose levels is believed to reduce the risk of development of long-term complications of diabetes. Early detection and treatment of established complications can reduce morbidity and costs.

For example, in retinopathy, the detection of early changes, followed by laser treatment, can prevent blindness. Planned follow-up with screening for complications is essential. Living with diabetes involves lifestyle modification to achieve optimal control of the condition. Time spent in listening, responding to questions and providing information and support is as essential to treatment as the prescription of diet, diet and medication, or diet and insulin.

The Diabetes Control and Complications Trial (DCCT), which was finished early in 1994, showed that greater efforts to control blood glucose levels led to a reduction in the risks of all the complications of diabetes. The study was only of those with type 1 diabetes, so transfer of these findings to type 2 diabetes cannot be made because of increased risks in the latter associated with tight glucose control in this group. A further study in the UK was carried out – UK Prospective Diabetes Study or UKPDS.

SUMMARY

- Diabetes is a common condition.
- With modern methods of treatment, people with diabetes can look forward to a near normal life.
- If treatment is less than optimal, acute illness may necessitate hospital admission. Complications affecting the eyes, kidneys and feet may seriously affect the quality of life.
- Diabetes can be costly to the patient and the NHS. Properly planned services and preventive activities can greatly reduce the cost to both.
- Present treatment of diabetes does not depend only on technology. An important aspect of care is the education of the patient and family.
- An important aspect of care is support and education.

The aims of diabetes care

The overall aims of any system of diabetes care are to facilitate diabetic self-management and control, enabling people with diabetes to make the necessary adjustments to remain well and happy, to reduce mortality, morbidity and hospitalisation, and to improve the early detection of complications by effective surveillance.

How is diabetes care organised in the UK?

In 2000, the Audit Commission identified that there was considerable variation in the standard of care provided for people with diabetes. Most districts have specialist diabetes clinics although these vary in quality. In some districts people with diabetes are followed up in general medical clinics. Increasingly, hospital clinics are being set up collaboratively for special problems. There may be joint clinics with obstetricians, joint renal clinics and foot clinics, including the expertise of vascular surgeons, chiropodists/podiatrists and orthotists (fitters of shoes and other appliances).

In many districts, clinics for children with diabetes are organised and run by a paediatrician with a special interest in diabetes. Out-of-hours peripheral clinics are available in some areas, providing a service for the adolescent and working populations.

About half the diabetic population regularly attend a hospital clinic with the specialist facilities this provides. Those attending the hospital are mainly the younger population (treated with diet and insulin) and those with established complications requiring particular surveillance and treatment.

The remaining 50% of the diabetic population are either cared for by their general practitioner and team or they receive no care at all. It is estimated that about 50% of general practices in the UK are providing an organised service of diabetes care. The remaining 50% of practices provide little or no care for their diabetic population.

On the whole interested general practitioners and their teams are looking after the type 2 diabetic population, where diabetes occurs in middle and later life. Often this type of diabetes has been regarded as 'mild'. This is not so. Type 2 diabetes affects 75% or more of the diabetic population; it is associated with all the complications of diabetes, which are not uncommonly already present at diagnosis.

The organisation of diabetes care is complex and ever-changing in the life of a person with diabetes, not only from the person's own perspective but also in the multitude of relatives and professionals who may be involved in his or her care, individually or collectively.

Support, education, good communications and an understanding of the availability of appropriate care by the person with diabetes, relatives and health care professionals are as important as the treatment of the condition.

The role of the specialist team

The specialist team in diabetes care has evolved over a number of years. The team includes:

- Physician/paediatrician
- Nurse specialist
- Dietitian
- Chiropodist/podiatrist.

The team may be extended under certain circumstances to include:

- Obstetrician
- Vascular surgeon
- Ophthalmologist
- Renal physician
- Psychologist.

The team should provide the expertise (based on training and experience) for the management of care of diabetes in the hospital setting and be available as a resource for care in the community.

The physician (diabetologist)

The physician:

- has a specialist *interest, training* and *experience* in the management of diabetes
- may have *research* interests
- is involved in the *leadership* of diabetes care in a district
- should be a *resource* for medical practitioners and health care professionals
- is dedicated to *raising awareness* of diabetes
- competes for *finance* and *resources* to support diabetes.

It is important that general practitioners and their teams providing diabetes care are aware of the physician(s) with a specialist interest in the district. Should problems arise, they will be quickly resolved where links have been established and communication is easy.

Many centres also have a paediatrician with a particular interest and training in the care of children and young people with diabetes. The paediatrician's team will consist of a nurse specialist (sometimes children trained) and a dietitian specialising in the needs of children.

Ideally, as children move towards adulthood, a collaborative service should be available where the paediatrician and physician caring for adults work together with appropriate teams to ensure that the change from childhood care to adult care is as smooth as possible.

The nurse specialist

The nurse specialist is a trained nurse with extended knowledge and skills in diabetes management as an educator, manager, researcher, communicator and innovator held responsible for his or her actions.

Diabetes nurse specialists work wholly in diabetes care, either full- or part-time with a physician(s) or paediatrician(s) involved in diabetes. The nurse may be based in a hospital or community but may visit in either depending on need. The nurse works either with adults or children with diabetes and their families, or with both. The nurse is a resource and adviser in diabetes for other health professionals in the health authority. The nurse specialist is an educator of colleagues in nursing and other disciplines in hospital and community and, working within the diabetes care team, provides the following services:

- A newly diagnosed person – help for the whole family in understanding and coming to terms with the condition.
- Stabilisation of people new to insulin.
- Understanding blood sugar control and how to monitor this. Advice on monitoring systems.
- Prevention of hypoglycaemia.
- Advice in the prevention and treatment of hyperglycaemia (e.g. during illness).
- Changing insulin regimens or insulin injection systems.
- Understanding and knowledge of diabetic complications.
- Prevention of foot problems.
- Education on all aspects of diabetes, individually or in groups for people with diabetes and colleagues.
- Support for the person with diabetes, the family and carers.
- Crisis management – in particular where there are psychological, social and family problems.
- Facilitating all aspects of diabetes care with appropriate health care professionals and others (e.g. teachers, employers).
- Providing the necessary expertise and materials or resources where requested or required.
- In association with other team members, the diabetes specialist nurse develops protocols, undertakes audit and sets standards.

Nurse specialists have incorporated into their job description the necessary authorisation for the alteration of insulin and medication in the treatment of diabetes. This authorisation is only provided with the agreement of the diabetologist or physician involved and after training in the management of diabetes by the nurse specialist. In addition, many nurse specialists provide an out-of-hours, weekend advisory service. It is well recognised that this is valued by people with diabetes, particularly by newly diagnosed people/children or their family/carers. A telephone call for advice may prevent an emergency situation arising.

The dietitian

The particular responsibilities of the dietitian in diabetes care include:

- Assessment of eating habits (individual and family).
- Advice on buying and cooking food.
- Ensuring adequate nutrition (especially in young and elderly people).

- Promoting healthy eating.
- Helping people to reduce weight.
- Stabilising weight.
- Meal planning (especially regular meals).
- Advice and planning of special dietary needs (e.g. for people in renal failure).

Interested dietitians are often involved in all aspects of diabetes support and education, to either individuals or groups. However, they may also be involved in the provision of other dietetic services. In general, dietitians are hospital based, working with their colleagues and linking in with the diabetologist and nurse specialist.

Community dietitians are spread thinly in the UK. Some districts do have them and they can be a valuable resource for dietetic advice in the community, in particular to general practice. In many districts, however, where no community dietitian is available, the person with diabetes is provided with dietetic advice by the practice nurse, district nurse, health visitor or general practitioner – often with very little training in the specific aspects of diabetic dietary requirements. It is the right of every person with diabetes to receive advice from a trained dietitian, who may be hospital based and is available in every district.

The dietitian should be an important resource in the provision of training and continuing education of all those providing diabetes care in the community. More community dietitians are required to meet this need.

The chiropodist/podiatrist

Within the NHS, each district provides a chiropody/podiatry service in community clinics and hospitals and at home for house-bound patients. Referrals come from doctors, nurses or patients themselves. Some hospitals and general practices provide chiropody within their diabetic clinics. The NHS employs only State-Registered Chiropodists (SRCh) who have trained for 3 years at one of the recognised schools. State-Registered Chiropodists also practise privately, as do unregistered chiropodists with varying amounts of training. Care should be taken therefore when referring people to a private chiropodist. Podiatrists are chiropodists with extended training.

Chiropody/podiatry services for people with diabetes. Both neuropathic and ischaemic ulcers are common in diabetic patients. The chiropodist has an important role in the teaching of all aspects of foot care, including advice about nail cutting and shoes to avoid the development of foot ulcers and about management of existing ulcers. A specialised multi-disciplinary foot clinic can halve the number of amputations in patients with diabetes as long as referral to these clinics is appropriate and in good time.

Most health authorities expect chiropodists to provide services for patients in four official priority groups:

- Senior citizens
- Children attending school
- Mentally or physically handicapped people
- Pregnant women.

Surprisingly, people with diabetes are not officially recognised as a priority group, but many chiropody/podiatry services do accept referrals of people with diabetes and other high-risk groups. At present most District Health Authorities do not purchase chiropody for otherwise well people between the ages of 16 and 65 years. Ideally, a range of foot problems should be officially recognised in the NHS. A more coherent policy is required, based on unmet need and its associated morbidity.

Chiropodists/podiatrists with an up-to-date knowledge of diabetes care have an important role in the prevention of disability in the management of diabetic foot problems. Their expertise includes:

- Assessment of foot structure and function
- The manufacture of orthoses (insoles, padding, special shoes)
- Advice on shoes/shoe fitting
- Ongoing surveillance
- Treatment (e.g. reduction of callus, nail care, débriding of ulcers).

A list of State-Registered Chiropodists employed by the health authority is available in every district, in headquarters or community units. Lists of private State-Registered Chiropodists are available in Yellow Pages. Fees for private chiropody services vary. Home visits are more costly than visits to a surgery.

Diabetes centres

Education of the person with diabetes and the family is a key factor in the reduction of morbidity and mortality, and the need for hospital admission. Improved education programmes may not only reduce the number of foot complications, but also drastically reduce admission rates for hypoglycaemia, ketoacidosis and the demands on accident and emergency departments, as well as achieving improvement in overall blood glucose control.

A hospital clinic is not the place for education programmes. Clinics may be large, busy and often staffed by inexperienced and frequently changing junior doctors. In an outpatient clinic, there are major obstacles to the success of education programmes, where time and skilled counselling may not be available and where the clinic environment is inappropriate.

The purpose of diabetes centres. There are many diabetes centres in the UK and more are planned.

The diabetes centre is a base for the specialist team and a focus for care provision and resources within the district. Its functions ideally include provision of:

- *A register* of all patients in the district in order to support hospital-based and general practitioner care systems and ensure adequate supervision or follow-up.
- *Appropriate organisation* and a pleasant environment for effective patient education (individually or in groups) which ensures the development and achievement of agreed objectives with:
  - ◆ primary education programmes for people with newly diagnosed diabetes (and their families/carers)
  - ◆ secondary education: long-term diabetes control counselling and maintenance and reinforcement of changes in behaviour
  - ◆ support for patients in hospital.
- *A communication centre* to:
  - ◆ provide a reference point for patient enquiries
  - ◆ ensure coordination between members of the diabetes team enabling the formulation and implementation of agreed objectives
  - ◆ provide integration with other hospital departments and staff to achieve common treatment policies
  - ◆ help general practitioner cooperative care schemes achieve common goals
  - ◆ act as a focal point for the training of medical and non-medical staff
  - ◆ streamline organisation and improve cost-effectiveness.
- *A comprehensive system of clinical care* and evaluation should ensure:
  - ◆ outpatient care of all new and follow-up patients
  - ◆ effective screening and surveillance procedures for complications
  - ◆ availability of facilities for treatment of diabetic complications and referral for non-diabetic medical problems
  - ◆ the development, maintenance and support of general practitioner cooperative care schemes.

Diabetes UK

The role of Diabetes UK in the organisation of diabetes care in the UK

Diabetes UK (formerly the British Diabetic Association, founded in 1934) has 140,000 members, mainly people with diabetes, those who care for them and health professionals, all with the common goal of improving care and quality of life for those with diabetes. Professional membership is organised into the Medical and Scientific section, and Education and Professional Care section and now the Primary Care of Diabetes (PCDUK) section. All meet regularly to exchange new information and ideas. Many clinicians with a special concern for diabetes are members and as a group have collected considerable data on many aspects of diabetes.

Diabetes UK also funds diabetes research. Of particular relevance is the UK Prospective Diabetes Study funded by the MRC, Diabetes UK and the pharmaceutical industry. This study aims to determine whether improved blood glucose control reduced complications in type 2 diabetes. This study has been in progress for over 10 years and should give important answers as to the best available treatment for type 2 diabetes in the near future.

Diabetes UK has an important role in any countrywide strategy for raising diabetes health care standards in the UK.

Diabetes UK is an important non-government organisation dedicated to raising awareness of diabetes and in attracting funds in order to support diabetes and research in the UK. It provides an authoritative source of information on living with diabetes to people with diabetes, those who care for them and health professionals. Activities include organising and contributing to scientific meetings and training courses, producing leaflets on specific topics and other educational material, seminars and conferences for lay people, and programmes for children and teenagers with diabetes. Information covers treatment, lifestyle, care and social aspects of diabetes. Diabetes UK's magazine *Balance* (readership around 250,000) is an important medium of communication countrywide. *Balance for Beginners* (editions for type 1 diabetes, type 2 diabetes, children and parents) is an important resource for people newly diagnosed with diabetes or those wanting an update. This is freely available on request to general practice clinics and individuals with diabetes/carers. Contact Diabetes UK (see resources list, Appendix VIII).

Services provided by Diabetes UK include:

- Diabetes care and information services
- Diet information services
- Youth department and family services
- Education services
- Primary Care Diabetes UK (PCDUK).

Diabetes care and information services

This department deals with questions relating to diabetes care from people with diabetes and their carers, and from health care professionals on any topic (e.g. insurance, driving, travel, benefits, aspects of care).

Diet information services

Dietitians and a home economist are available to provide dietary advice and suggestions for healthy eating and meal planning as well as creating recipes. These are available in published form – see Appendix VIII for details.

Youth and family services

The Youth department provides services for children and young people with diabetes from the onset of their diabetes to the age of 25 years (and for anyone else involved with them: parents, teachers, careers officers and others). They run holiday and activity courses throughout the UK for children aged 5–18. Family weekends are run from October to April. Youth packs and school packs are also provided by this department.

Education services

Deals with the educational aspects of all Diabetes UK's activities, whether for health care professionals or lay people.

Professional sections

These include Medical and Scientific sections, Education and Care sections and PCDUK (see Appendix IV).

Branches of Diabetes UK

There are over 400 local branches of Diabetes UK across Britain and Northern Ireland. They are all run by volunteers with support from the local area coordinator and a volunteer. A contact list is available comprising: parent groups (young people with diabetes), youth diabetes groups, self-help groups, Asian support groups, groups for the visually impaired as well as ordinary branches who have regular meetings. The whole of this voluntary section is coordinated at its Queen Anne Street office in London where information can be obtained regarding local groups. Contact the Voluntary Groups section. There are currently two regional offices in the north-west of England and in Scotland. Further regional offices are planned.

Funding of Diabetes UK

Diabetes UK is funded by voluntary contributions; no government funding is provided. One particular countrywide event that takes place every year during

June is National Diabetes Week. During this, local branch members are involved in house-to-house collections and can be seen in high streets.

The Information Department

The Information Department provides a database for health care professionals providing bibliographies and a bi-monthly list of all relevant publications. Contact Diabetes UK (see resources list, Appendix VIII).

Further reading

Diabetes UK produce a whole range of magazines, leaflets and books. Contact them for a catalogue.

Audit Commission (2000). *Testing Times: A review of diabetes services in England and Wales.* London: Audit Commission.

British Diabetic Association (1995). *Your Child and Diabetes.* Balance for Beginners format.

British Diabetic Association (1995). *Pregnancy, Diabetes and You.* London: BDA.

British Diabetic Association (1995). *Diabetes in the United Kingdom – 1996.* London: BDA.

Consumers Association (1991). What chiropody offers. *Drug and Therapeutics Bulletin* 29(8): 29–30.

Day JL, Spathis M (1988). District diabetes centres in the United Kingdom. Workshop report. *Diabetic Medicine* 5: 372–80.

DCCT (1993). The effect of intensive treatment of diabetes on the development and progression of long-term complications in insulin-dependent diabetes mellitus. *New England Journal of Medicine* 329: 977–86.

Diabetes UK. *Balance.* Issued bi-monthly.

Diabetes UK. *Diabetes for Beginners (Type 1).* London: Diabetes UK.

Diabetes UK. *Diabetes for Beginners (Type 2).* London: Diabetes UK.

Diabetes UK (2001). Diabetes UK Report 'Missing Million'. London, Diabetes UK.

Haw N, Thompson AV, Thorogood M, Fowler GH, Mann JI (1989). Diabetes in the elderly: the Oxford Community Diabetes Study. *Diabetic Medicine* 6: 608–13.

Joint Working Party on Diabetic Renal Failure of the British Diabetic Association, The Renal Association and The Research Unit of the Royal College of Physicians (1988). Renal failure in diabetes in the UK: deficient provision of care in 1985. *Diabetic Medicine* 5: 79–84.

Marks L (1996). *Counting the Cost: The Real Impact of Non-insulin-dependent Diabetes.* London: King's Fund/BDA.

Murphy M (1991). *The Health of the Nation. Response from the British Diabetic Association.* London: British Diabetic Association.

Royal College of Nursing Diabetes Nursing Forum Document (1991). *The Role of the Specialist Nurse.* London: Royal College of Nursing.

Tunbridge WMG (1981). Factors contributing to deaths of diabetics underpay years of age. *The Lancet* ii: 569–72.

UK Prospective Diabetes Study IV (1988). Characteristics of newly presenting type 2 diabetic patients: male preponderance and obesity at different ages. *Diabetic Medicine* 5: 154–9.

UKPDS 33. *Lancet* 1998; 352: 837–53.

UKPDS 34. *Lancet* 1998; 352: 854–65.

UKPDS 35. *BMJ* 2000; 321: 405–12.

UKPDS 36. *BMJ* 2000; 321: 412–19.

UKPDS 38. *BMJ* 1998; 317: 703–13.

UKPDS 39. *BMJ* 1998; 317: 713–20.

Watkins PJ, Drury PL, Howell SL (1996). *Diabetes and Its Management,* 5th edn. Oxford: Blackwell Science.

Part II

Providing diabetes care

4 The diabetes service in general practice

- How to set up a system of care
- Planning the service
- Provision of the service: day, time and frequency
- Essential equipment
- Materials/resources for diabetes education

How to set up a system of care

Aims

1. *To identify, know* and *register* the diabetes population covered by the practice.
2. *To provide treatment, support, education* and *surveillance* for people with diabetes not receiving hospital care or where care is 'shared' or 'integrated'. (For definition of 'shared/integrated care' for people with diabetes, see pages 48–9.)
3. *To know and use all available specialist and support services* – referring to these in good time and appropriately.

Objectives

1. Planning and organisation of registration, recall and follow-up systems and their regular update.
2. A planned programme of care for all those receiving the practice diabetes service including:
   (a) initial support, assessment and treatment of newly diagnosed people with diabetes including immediate referral for specialist services, where appropriate
   (b) initial and staged continuing education that is correct, consistent and up to date

(c) planned appropriate treatment (taking into account age, lifestyle, knowledge and understanding), which achieves the maintenance of near normal blood glucose control

(d) management of acute complications (such as hyperglycaemia, ketosis and hypoglycaemia)

(e) identification of risk factors for long-term effects of diabetes, such as:
    (i) hypertension
    (ii) hyperlipidaemia

(f) early identification, surveillance, treatment (and referral, if appropriate) of long-term complications of diabetes in order to reduce:
    (i) blindness and visual impairment
    (ii) foot ulceration, limb amputation disability
    (iii) end-stage renal failure
    (iv) premature ill health and early death resulting from the macrovascular complications of ischaemic heart disease, peripheral vascular disease and cerebrovascular disease.

Planning the service

Careful planning by the practice team involves the following:

■ Knowledge of the practice diabetes population in terms of numbers, type of diabetes (treatment) and who is currently providing their care.

■ Organisation of the service (in relation to other services provided by the practice).

■ Availability of the necessary skills.

■ Identification of training or continuing education requirements by members of the team involved.

■ Necessary equipment, education material and resources required (other than those currently available in the practice).

■ Methods of record keeping to be employed.

■ Planning the start date for the service in relation to the necessary preparation period.

Involvement and discussion by members of the team will identify possible organisational problems and resource implications early. It may be helpful for a member of the local hospital specialist team or specialist facilitator to be invited to the practice during the planning period. This would have the following advantages:

- Establishing a relationship and communication between the practice and the hospital diabetes team.
- Signifying the practice's intentions and plans for their service so that the specialist team is aware of them.
- Providing awareness of the available local and national diabetes specialist and support facilities.
- Setting up the necessary links for sharing care.
- Discussion around diabetes management and local protocols for care, criteria for referral and mechanisms for urgent referral (such as a newly diagnosed child with diabetes or a person with foot ulceration).
- Training or updating requirements by the team to be involved in the practice diabetes service.

Planning the service will also involve consideration of dietetic, chiropody and perhaps counselling services. Depending on district services available, the practice may decide to provide these 'in house'.

It is important that, if expertise is acquired by the practice in these areas, the professionals employed are qualified (i.e. State-Registered Dietitians and State-Registered Chiropodists) and that they have an up-to-date knowledge of current diabetes management.

The planning period should also encompass plans for the ongoing review of the diabetes service and consideration of its evaluation and annual audit. It is also a useful time for discussion with local services (such as pharmacists, opticians) to raise awareness regarding the proposed diabetes service.

Finally, and most importantly, the preparation time before the commencement of the service should include discussion about diabetes, identifying any problems that members of the team may have in the future provision of a high-quality service for people with diabetes in the care of the practice.

Organisation of the service

Practices vary in their organisation of diabetes care; often the system employed relates to the size of practice.

Small practices with one general practitioner may have only 20 people identified with diabetes. If a third or a half of these receive care provided by the hospital services, the number cared for in the practice is small, perhaps not warranting even a monthly clinic. Such a practice may provide a service to individuals within surgery time. Some general practitioners may prefer this, so long as there is an established recall system and there is enough time during the consultation to provide an adequate service. In larger practices, a regular 'diabetes' clinic may be required within protected time.

The advantage of 'protected' time in a diabetes clinic is that the focus at that time is on diabetes care. People with diabetes attending the practice are aware that the diabetes clinic is on a certain day at the same time, and regular attendance becomes routine. However, it is important that people unable to attend such a 'clinic' because of work or other commitments can be offered the service at other times. Organising a service that is flexible also encourages attendance.

Another group who need to be identified are people with diabetes who are housebound and unable to attend the surgery, and not receiving diabetes care and surveillance from the hospital or any other health care provider. District nurses are involved in diabetes care for those who are dependent for their care in the short or long term. The care provided by district nurses is usually related to treatment – the administration of insulin, foot/leg dressings or supervision of these, and monitoring diabetes control. There is more integration in some practices, e.g. district nurse using record cards to record reviews. Management of diabetes and surveillance for problems and detection of complications in the housebound diabetic individuals will need inclusion in the organisation of the practice service by the team involved. The district nurse or practice nurse should visit the housebound diabetic individuals regularly, discussing care with the general practitioner who will provide a follow-up visit periodically and at least an annual review.

Who might be offered the practice diabetes service?

In every district, it is to be hoped that discussions will have been held between specialist teams and general practitioners as to the arrangements for diabetes care provision and suggested criteria for referral and sharing care.

The service could be offered to the following:

- People with type 2 diabetes.
- Some people with type 1 diabetes.
- People with diabetes wishing to attend the practice for their care.
- Those who are very elderly or frail for whom hospital care is inappropriate unless absolutely essential.
- Those who are housebound.
- Those discharged from hospital care or where no care provision is identified.
- Those attending hospital for other conditions, where diabetes care, education and surveillance are not provided by other specialists.

Who will be involved in the provision of the practice diabetes service?

A minimum team, in a moderate to large practice, would consist of a receptionist/secretary, nurse and doctor. In a large practice more than one receptionist/secretary and nurse may be required to keep the service and its administration running throughout the year. In a practice where many doctors may be in partnership, which doctor(s) will be involved requires clarification at an early stage. In some practices all the medical practitioners wish to be involved in the total care of their own patients. This system is feasible, so long as the person running the service (e.g. the nurse) communicates with each doctor about the care of each patient. The argument put forward in favour of this system is that all the medical practitioners retain their skill in the management of diabetes.

However, a disadvantage of this system is that all the doctors may not be able to retain their knowledge and skills with very few patients to manage. It is therefore probably best, in the interests of a quality service, for one doctor in the practice to take overall responsibility for diabetes care. Continuing education and the management of many patients will ensure retention of knowledge and skills. This doctor can provide the necessary leadership for the diabetes service, at the same time communicating with colleagues about the service and the progress of their individual patients. Further, the identified team will provide continuity and consistency of information – important in diabetes care where conflicting messages are often received by people with diabetes in their dealings with many health care professionals.

The nurse's role is also important in continuity of care, in the support and education of clerks and reception staff, and in communicating with the doctors in the practice and other providers of care.

Provision of the service: day, time and frequency

In order to decide on the best day, time and how often the service will be provided, the following should be considered:

- Numbers of people with diabetes (see page 23).
- Those requiring practice diabetes care.
- Those requiring shared/integrated care (see pages 48–9).
- Organisation for patients usually attending a branch surgery (perhaps more than one, especially in rural areas).
- Primary health services already offered by the practice.
- Availability of medical, nursing and administration time.
- Appropriate and available facilities (rooms, storage of equipment, educational materials).
- Transport services, especially for those who are visually impaired or disabled.
- Organisation for annual review, where eye screening may be arranged as a separate session(s) annually.

- Availability and timing of laboratory collections (e.g. venous blood taken for measurement of glycated haemoglobin should be collected the same day or stored in the refrigerator and collected no later than the next day).
- Sufficient time for individual patient care and education at a routine appointment (at least 20 minutes) and at annual review (at least 30 minutes). More time may be required.
- Identified time within the clinic for administration, record keeping and individual follow-up care that may be required for individual patients (e.g. arranging for chiropody, obtaining advice from a diabetes team, enquiring about appropriate social services benefits).
- Extra time or 'leeway' of time should be available for:
  - new patients to the practice
  - people with newly diagnosed diabetes
  - those with diabetes requiring urgent care or advice for a specific problem which cannot or should not be left until the next scheduled appointment.

Numbers of people with diabetes

In a large practice where numbers may be high (perhaps as a result of an older population) or the ethnic composition is high (e.g. Asians from the subcontinent of India or south Asians; African–Caribbeans), it may be necessary to hold a clinic every week. In a small practice, a clinic may only be required monthly or even bi-monthly.

Shared care (integrated care)

> **In the management of diabetes, the provision of care should aim to be organised and individual to the person concerned. During the lifetime of a person with diabetes, care is provided by the primary care team or a specialist team, or both. The appropriate care provider will change according to the progress of the condition, the need for optimum management and the wishes of the person with diabetes.**

Where care is 'shared' or 'integrated' it is important that each provider is aware of the other in the diabetes management and that the person with diabetes understands the nature of the care provided by primary care and specialist teams.

In 'integrated' care, good communication and record keeping by all providers are essential. A person care card (cooperation card) held by the person with diabetes may be useful so long as it is filled in by all those concerned!

Care provision (who does what, where and when) is an important part of diabetes education for all people with diabetes.

Finally, it is important that 'integrated' care is understood by all concerned – with each individual person with diabetes. Where these demarcations do not exist, care may be duplicated or not provided at all.

Ideal facilities for the diabetes service

There are no special facilities necessary for diabetes care other than those that would be provided for all primary health care.

Consideration should be given to flexible use of the waiting area, perhaps for periodic educational group sessions when discussions can be held and videos shown. This area may also be used for the display of literature about diabetes and information regarding local services and facilities along with other health care educational material.

No particular clinical room facilities are necessary, other than a dark room, where fundoscopy examination will take place, and space for the correct distance to be measured between the patient and the Snellen chart (for testing vision). A six metre distance and chart are commonly used, although in a small surgery a three metre chart can be obtained or a six metre chart used with a mirror (see section on testing for visual acuity in Chapter 10).

Who does what in which room is often a cause for debate! Where the nurse and doctor are setting up a new service, it may be helpful for both to work together in one room until confidence is gained and each understands the other's role. Later, the organisation may change to clinical checks and education provided by the nurse, a review of these by the doctor with further medical checks, discussion and prescription to complete the periodic or annual review and the follow-up care decided appropriately.

It should be remembered that people with diabetes attending the surgery or medical centre may be elderly, visually impaired or disabled, and any facilities for diabetes care should accommodate these problems.

Essential equipment

General

Hand-washing facilities with warm water, soap and paper towels
Important for finger-prick tests for blood glucose levels and good hygiene.

Weighing scales (metric or imperial)
These should be checked and calibrated annually.

Weight conversion chart (kilograms to stones/pounds)
Available from visiting pharmaceutical representatives.

'Ideal' weight chart
That is, weight for height (i.e. the body mass index or BMI) of men and women (available from pharmaceutical representatives).

Height gauge
Correctly positioned to record correct height.

Equipment for collection of laboratory samples
For example, blood, urine, wound swabs.

Sphygmomanometer with standard cuff
Small and large cuffs should also be available and these should be checked annually. (3M Health Care Ltd provides a FREE service – see resources list, Appendix VIII.)

Disposable gloves

Sharps disposal container

Screening and monitoring

Note: multiple urine test strips are available, although expensive (Boehringer Mannheim and Bayer plc).

Clock or wrist watch with second hand
Essential for the correct timing of urine and capillary blood tests.

White cotton wool/tissues for removal of blood from test strips
Coloured cotton wool/tissues should not be used as they may affect results. Cotton wool/tissues are not necessary with non-wipe test strips.

Screening

For glucose and protein in the urine
Strips such as Uristix (Bayer plc) are required as well as measurement of blood glucose if glycosuria is found. Occasionally an oral glucose tolerance test (OGTT) is necessary (see section 'Screening for diabetes mellitus' in Chapter 5).

Lucozade 375 ml or 75 g glucose for OGTT
Glucose may be obtained on prescription if the patient is exempt from charges, otherwise it is cheaper (than paying a prescription charge) to buy ready measured from the pharmacy (see section 'Oral glucose tolerance test' in Chapter 5).

Monitoring

Urine testing

For glucose in the urine (quantitative)
Diastix and Clinistix (Bayer plc) or Diabur Test 5000 (Roche Diagnostics).
Note: ketones may inhibit colour change in Diastix.

For protein in the urine (quantitative)
Albustix (Bayer plc).

For microalbuminuria
Micral Test (Roche Diagnostics – strips) or Microalbumin Test (Bayer plc – tablets).

For ketones in the urine
Ketostix and Ace Test (Bayer plc) or Ketur Test (Roche Diagnostics). For use in illness (and on diagnosis).

Capillary blood testing

Finger-pricking devices/lancets for multiple use
Softclix pro (mulitiple blood sampler) and Safe-T-pro (single-use device) (Roche Diagnostics); Autolet Mini, Autolet Lite and Autolet Clinisafe Lite (Owen Mumford); Microlet (Bayer plc).
Note: lancets are available on FP10, although lancets for multiple use are not available on FP10. Finger-pricking devices can be purchased or are available via hospital prescription.

Test strips for blood glucose measurement
BM-Test 1-44 Sticks (Roche Diagnostics). Glucostix (Bayer plc) and Glucotide (Bayer plc) for use with Glucometer 4. All available on FP10. Bayer plc do not sell Glucometer 4; their glucose meter is the Esprit meter.

A further strip that provides visual proof only (no actual reading): Medi-Test (BHR). Supreme (Hypoguard) can be used as visual proof or for meter.

Blood glucose meters and test strips
Appropriate to the meter used.

Note: meters are not essential (even though they may be given away free). If the practice is given or purchases a meter, care should be taken to calibrate it with the correct strips and quality control solution used to monitor the accuracy of the instrument.

Testing for peripheral neuropathy

Patella hammer
For checking reflexes.

Tuning fork
For checking vibration sensation (CO 128).

Monofilaments (neurotips)
Monofilaments and neurotips are used for checking lower limb sensation. Cotton wool/pin can be used if monofilaments are not available.

Checking visual acuity

Snellen chart
Well lit.

Measuring tape
To mark distance on floor for patient to view chart (six metres for six metre chart, three metres for three metre chart; if a mirror is used with a three metre chart in a small space, a three metre distance should be marked for viewing the chart).

Pinhole card
To be held in front of the eye by the patient to discount errors of refraction, should visual acuity be reduced.

Fundoscopy: screening for diabetic retinopathy

Ophthalmoscope
With spare bulb and charged batteries (regular checking required).

Mydriatic drops
For dilating pupils, e.g. tropicamide 0.5–1%.

For emergency use: for the treatment of hypoglycaemia

In surgery	**In doctor's bag**
Lucozade/glucose tablets	Hypostop gel
Hypostop gel (available on FP10)	IMI glucagon
IMI glucagon (available on FP10)	Intravenous dextrose
Blood glucose measuring strips	Blood glucose measuring strips

Materials/resources for diabetes education

Resources and/or educational materials are available from drug companies (see Appendix VIII). The local diabetes team can also help to recommend appropriate literature. See also Chapter 13, 'Education for self-management'.

The first five items are often available from pharmaceutical companies (see resources list, Appendix VIII, for addresses).

Posters
Give information. Useful as educational aids on specific topics.

Information booklets/leaflets
For individual and appropriate use.

Videos
For education sessions.

Self-monitoring diaries

Identification cards

Multimedia
Diabetes education programmes.

Local diabetes units/centres
Contact numbers.

Diabetes UK
Local branches for adults and parent groups – contact numbers.

Local information and contact numbers

- Chiropody (podiatry) services
- Dietetic services
- Dental services
- Pharmacy services
- Optician services
- Supporting/caring agencies/trusts
- Social services and benefits
- Rehabilitation services.

Further information
This may be required for:

- Shopping (e.g. specific foods, shoe fitting)
- Leisure facilities
- Travel/holidays (e.g. immunisation).

Materials for organisation and recording information

- Diabetes register
- Recall sheet/card index $\big\}$ perhaps held on computer.
- Appointment cards – for patient use.
- Appointment book – to record appointments made.
- Standard letter – for use for new patients attending and recall.
- Card/leaflet – with practice information and practice contact numbers.
- Laboratory forms.
- Patient's medical records.
- Diabetes record of care (held by the person with diabetes or the practice; perhaps held on computer).
- Minimum data set (agreed locally) – see Chapter 15, p. 215, 'Monitoring and audit' of practice diabetes care.

Recording information

Individual diabetes record of care (Fig. 4.1)

- Every person with diabetes should have their care recorded. This should include at least:
  - ◆ demographic information
  - ◆ a record of clinical checks and results
  - ◆ a record of education topics covered

- ◆ a record of treatment targets and management
- ◆ a record of particular problems and actions taken (or to be taken).
- ■ Where the information is to be recorded requires discussion and a practice decision. The options might be:
  - ◆ information recorded on computer – printed out – practice medical record (this will make the medical records bulky); *note:* it is necessary for a written record of care to be made for medicolegal purposes
  - ◆ information recorded in practice medical records
  - ◆ information recorded in Diabetes Record Card (practice held)
  - ◆ information recorded in Diabetes Record Card (patient held) and in practice medical records or in Diabetes Record Card (practice held).
- ■ Should any problem or question arise regarding the care of a patient, the diabetes record is the only demonstration of care provided (particularly if care is only provided by the practice).

Fig. 4.1 Example of a practice-held record card. A template for a patient-held record card is reproduced in Appendix IX, page 301

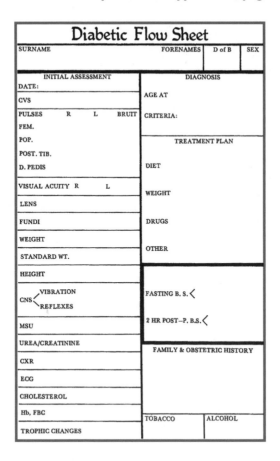

■ Diabetes Record (cooperation) Cards may be:
- ◆ provided by the district
- ◆ provided by pharmaceutical companies (e.g. Boehringer Mannheim)
- ◆ designed by individual practices for their own use.

Practice information relating to diabetes care provision

In order to assess the health needs of the practice population and for the short- and long-term planning of the practice diabetes service, the recording of information is necessary for the following reasons:

■ To monitor the diabetes service.
■ To evaluate diabetes care provided.
■ To obtain statistical information (e.g. epidemiological, medical – see Chapter 15).

5   The symptoms of diabetes mellitus

> ■ Public awareness of diabetes
> ■ Screening for diabetes mellitus
> ■ Diagnosis of diabetes mellitus
> ■ Identification of people with diabetes mellitus
> ■ The practice diabetes register

The symptoms of diabetes are similar in both types of the condition. There are, however, certain differences between type 1 diabetes and type 2 diabetes. The two most important to remember are:

1. The rate of onset of symptoms:
   (a) fast in type 1 diabetes
   (b) slow in type 2 diabetes.
2. (a) Symptoms may be present but unrecognised in type 2 diabetes by the patient or the physician.
   (b) Presenting symptoms in type 1 diabetes are more obvious to the patient but may not always be recognised by the physician.

Increased awareness of diabetes in general practice has led to earlier diagnosis of type 1 diabetes, possibly before the patient is acutely ill; however, this has led to occasional misdiagnosis, with people being completely inappropriately treated as having type 2 diabetes, treated with diet alone, then given tablets, with no insulin being started until the person is acutely ill. It cannot be emphasised sufficiently that, if patient is under 35, thin already (particularly if athletic), then **think type 1 diabetes** even if the symptoms are not acute.

Table 5.1 shows the symptoms of diabetes as they occur in type 1 and type 2 diabetes, and the similarities and differences between the two types of condition.

Table 5.1 The symptoms of diabetes mellitus

Symptoms	Type 1 diabetes	Type 2 diabetes
Onset	Fast (weeks)	Slow (months, years)
Thirst	✓	✓
Polyuria/nocturia	✓	✓
Incontinence in elderly people	—	✓
Bed wetting in children	✓	—
Tiredness/lethargy	✓	✓
Mood changes (irritability)	✓	✓
Weight loss	✓++	✓
Visual disturbances	✓	✓
Thrush infections (genital)	✓	✓
Recurrent infections (boils/ulcers)	✓	✓
Hunger	✓	✓
Tingling/pain/numbness (in feet, legs, hands)	—	✓
Occasionally, abdominal pain	✓	—
Unexplained symptoms	✓	✓

The signs of diabetes (i.e. those that can be measured) are shown in Table 5.2, based on the WHO diagnostic criteria for 2000. The presence or absence of glycosuria, ketonuria, fasting and random blood glucose levels for the diagnosis of diabetes can be seen.

Table 5.2 Signs of diabetes mellitus (that can be measured)

Signs	Type 1 diabetes	Type 2 diabetes
Glycosuria	Present	May be absent
Fasting blood glucose	Venous or capillary whole blood ≥ 7.0 mmol/1	
Random blood glucose	Venous or capillary whole blood ≥ 11.1 mmol/1	
Ketonuria	May be present	Usually absent

Public awareness of diabetes

Symptoms and signs of type 1 diabetes are usually acute and the diagnosis should be made quickly, once the patient or family seeks advice.

Many people with type 2 diabetes live with the condition undiagnosed for months or years before seeking advice, by which time complications are well established.

The general public may well know 'something' about diabetes. This is often that diabetes is associated with 'sugar'. The nature of the association, however, is not necessarily understood. More importantly, the symptoms are not known or, because of their non-specific nature, are not related to the diagnosis of diabetes.

Symptoms of tiredness or lethargy may be explained away by 'I'm getting older', irritability by stress at work or in the home. Repeated infections may be treated by different doctors in a large practice and the significance of their frequency not realised. Symptoms may also occur or progress so slowly and in such a 'mild' way that they are not connected to type 2 diabetes.

Improving public awareness of diabetes

- All members of the public are registered with a doctor (or should be). The primary care team in the practice should always have 'diabetes' in their thoughts when providing any health care.
- Posters (Fig. 5.1) can be put up in surgeries and waiting areas showing the symptoms of diabetes.
- Health questionnaires used in routine screening or for new patients to the

practice should contain questions about symptoms of diabetes (as shown in the sample poster – Fig. 5.1).

Fig. 5.1 Poster showing symptoms of diabetes – for surgery use

DIABETES – DO YOU SUFFER FROM

- Excessive thirst?
- Going to the toilet to pass water (a lot)?
- Visual changes?
- Genital irritation?

- Lethargy?
- Weight loss?
- Mood changes?
- Weight gain?

IF SO PLEASE LET US KNOW

Screening for diabetes mellitus

Mass screening for the detection of diabetes entails considerable organisation and costs. However, screening of certain groups of people at risk is feasible and cost effective. An opportunistic, routine or 'on suspicion' approach should be adopted.

The following gives a good idea of who should be screened, who could be screened and the opportunities available for screening.

When opportunities for screening (by the primary health care team) can present
- During surgery
- In health promotion clinics
- When new patients present to the practice
- At 'home' screening programmes, e.g. with elderly people
- At routine medical checks, e.g. for insurance purposes.

People who should be screened (those with the following symptoms)
- Thirst
- Polyuria/nocturia
- Bed wetting in children

- Incontinence in elderly people
- Weight loss (sudden or gradual)
- Lethargy
- Mood changes
- Persistent infections (boils, abscesses, slow healing ulcers)
- Visual changes
- Symptoms of neuropathy/pins and needles in the feet and legs
- Unexplained symptoms.

People who could be screened (those more likely to develop diabetes)
- People with a family history (of diabetes mellitus)
- Overweight people
- Elderly people
- Asians from Indian subcontinent/African–Caribbeans
- Pregnant women
- Women with obstetric history (babies > 4 kg; unexplained fetal loss)
- People with peripheral vascular disease
- People with cardiac problems
- People with circulatory problems.

Diagnosis of diabetes mellitus

Important notes

Confirmation of urine test – positive for glucose

Should a urine test reveal the presence of glucose, it is important that further tests are carried out for fasting and/or random blood glucose levels (or by oral glucose tolerance test), as glycosuria may be the result of a *low* renal threshold.

Conversely, the diagnosis of diabetes may be missed in an older person with a HIGH renal threshold (the urine test may show a *negative* result, where the blood glucose level is 13 mmol/1 or more).

The renal threshold

The renal threshold (Fig. 5.2) is the level at which glucose spills over into the urine as blood glucose levels rise. A normal renal threshold is about 10 mmol/l (i.e. when the blood glucose level is measured, it is 10 mmol/l and glycosuria is detectable). The renal threshold usually rises with age so that high blood

Fig. 5.2 The renal threshold

1. **Normal renal threshold**

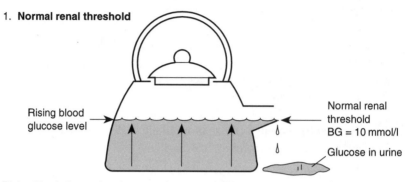

Rising blood glucose level → ← Normal renal threshold BG = 10 mmol/l

Glucose in urine

Rising blood glucose levels cause glucose to spill into urine at 10 mmol/l.

2. **High renal threshold**

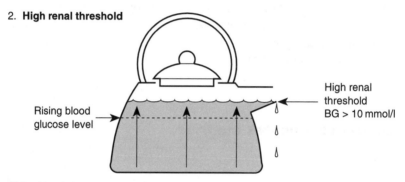

High renal threshold BG > 10 mmol/l

Rising blood glucose level →

Rising blood glucose levels may not show in urine.

3. **Low renal threshold**

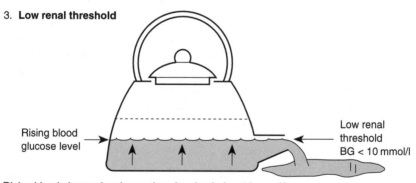

Rising blood glucose level →

← Low renal threshold BG < 10 mmol/l

Rising blood glucose level may show in urine below 10 mmol/l.

glucose levels are present in the absence of glycosuria. The renal threshold may be low in some people and particularly during pregnancy (Fig. 5.2).

Telling the patient

Once glycosuria has been found, the patient should be told of this and that further tests are required for the following reasons:

- The patient may not have diabetes but may have a low renal threshold (e.g. in pregnancy).
- The patient has diabetes (if pregnant – gestational diabetes).
- The patient has impaired glucose tolerance (IGT).
- The patient has impaired fasting glycaemia.

Reassurance of the patient is important and confirmation of the diagnosis should be made as quickly as possible so that appropriate treatment, support and education can begin. Preconceived ideas, fear and anxiety surround a diagnosis of diabetes. Firm evidence and careful explanation are essential, whether a diagnosis is confirmed or not.

Confirming the diagnosis

It has never been easy to classify and diagnose diabetes mellitus, because its very heterogeneity and characteristics have rendered most attempts at subdivision not entirely accurate and unable to reflect its underlying nature. There were anomalies in the earliest classification by age of onset and the replacement by pathogenic mechanism (type 1 or type 2 diabetes, IGT), which was linked to treatment, also caused confusion and uncertainty. New WHO diagnostic criteria were ratified in 2000.

The diagnosis of diabetes should be confirmed by diabetes symptoms plus a **random laboratory venous plasma glucose concentration of ≥ 11.1 mmol/l or a fasting plasma glucose concentration of ≥ 7.0 mmol/l or a 2-hour plasma glucose concentration of ≥ 11.1 mmol/l 2 hours after 75 g anhydrous glucose in an oral glucose tolerance test (OGTT).**

The hearty breakfast test

If the patient attends the surgery after an overnight fast, a laboratory venous sample (for blood glucose) can be obtained. After this, a 'hearty breakfast' (see box on page 64) is eaten (at home by the patient!) followed by a second laboratory venous blood sample (for blood glucose) taken 2 hours later.

A hearty breakfast menu

- Fruit juice
- Cereal and milk (with sugar if taken)
- Coffee or tea (with sugar if taken)
- Cooked breakfast (eggs, bacon, etc. if liked)
- Toast and marmalade

Note: an alternative to the 'hearty breakfast' would be 375 ml of Lucozade (supplied by the patient) and a venous blood sample taken 2 hours later.

Impaired glucose tolerance

Impaired glucose tolerance (IGT) is indicated by a fasting plasma glucose of < 7.0 mmol/l. Confirmation of IGT is made by the performance of an oral glucose tolerance test (OGTT): 2-hour value ≥ 7.8 mmol/l but < 11.1 mmol/l.

Impaired fasting glycaemia

Impaired fasting glycaemia (IFG) has been introduced to classify individuals who have fasting glucose values above the normal range but below those diagnostic of diabetes: fasting plasma glucose of ≥ 6.1 mmol/l but < 7.0 mmol/l. Diabetes UK recommends that all those with IFG should have an OGTT to exclude the diagnosis of diabetes. They are actively managed with lifestyle advice. If the glucose remains elevated above 6 mmol/l after at least 3 months, treatment with an oral hypoglycaemic agent should be considered, in the light of the UKPDS findings.

Oral glucose tolerance test (OGTT)
Local policy about this test varies, and in some areas the tests are carried out only by the local laboratory on venous blood, not on capillary blood sampling with use of surgery meters.

WHO recommendation. The OGTT is used principally for diagnosis when blood glucose levels are doubtful, during pregnancy, or to screen for diabetes and impaired glucose tolerance or impaired fasting glycaemia in an epidemiological setting.

The test
- The test should be administered in the morning, following at least three days of unrestricted diet (greater than 150 g of carbohydrate daily, i.e. full

daily meals and snacks including bread and potatoes) and usual physical activities.

- The test should be preceded by an overnight fast (10–16 hours) during which water may be drunk.
- Smoking is not permitted during the test.
- Factors influencing interpretation of the test should be recorded (e.g. infection, inactivity, medications).
- A fasting venous blood sample should be collected first. 'Fasting' and the time should be noted on the accompanying form.
- The patient is then given 75 g of glucose in 250–300 ml of water (PLJ – lemon juice – may make this more palatable, as patients often find the glucose solution nauseating). Alternatively, 375 ml Lucozade may be used. The glucose solution or Lucozade should be taken over approximately 5 minutes. The drink is more palatable taken through a straw.
- A venous blood sample should be taken 2 hours after the glucose load (samples may also be taken at half-hourly intervals during this period, for a more detailed profile).
- The accompanying laboratory form(s) should state the time of the glucose load and the collection time of the blood sample.
- Samples should be sent straight to the laboratory following completion of the test.
- Results will vary according to whether whole blood or plasma, venous or capillary samples are used.

Summary

For a summary see Tables 5.3 and 5.4.

Table 5.3 Glucose values for diabetes: random sample

	Diabetes likely	Diabetes uncertain	Diabetes unlikely
Venous plasma (mmol/l)	≥ 11.1	5.5–< 11.1	< 5.5
Venous blood (mmol/l)	≥ 10.0	4.4–< 10.0	< 4.4
Capillary plasma (mmol/l)	≥ 12.2	5.5–< 12.2	< 5.5
Capillary blood (mmol/l)	≥ 11.1	4.4–< 11.1	< 4.4

Source: Bodansky J (1994). In *Pocket Picture Guides. Diabetes*, 2nd edition. Fig 1. London: Wolfe Publishing

Table 5.4 Standardised oral glucose tolerance test

	Diabetes (mmol/1)	IGT (mmol/1)	IFG (mmol/1)
Venous			
Plasma			
fasting	≥ 7.0	< 7.0	≥ 6.1 – ≤ 7.0
2 hours	≥ 11.1	≥ 7.8–< 11.1	
Whole blood			
fasting	≥ 6.1	–	
2 hours	≥ 11.1	–	

IFG (impaired fasting glycaemia): new category (2000) which classifies individuals who have fasting glucose values above the normal range, but below those diagnostic of diabetes. Diabetes UK (2000).

Identification of people with diabetes mellitus

Details of people newly diagnosed with diabetes should be noted on a register (computer or written), as should those identified with diabetes and new to the practice. People attending the practice who are already diagnosed with diabetes can be identified through records, prescriptions and at surgery attendance. Medical notes should be flagged following identification as (Diab).

Those treated with diet alone or who are housebound are more difficult to identify as they may not collect prescriptions or require, or be able, to attend the surgery for health care services.

Compiling a list

■ Practice staff and the primary care team need to 'think diabetes'!
■ Administrative staff (clerks/receptionists) should be educated about diabetes so that they can recognise the names of test strips, drugs and insulin on prescriptions and identify people from their treatment and monitoring strips.
■ A 'named' person should be given responsibility for the list. This person can also remind others in the practice to note names of people with diabetes seen in surgery, health promotion clinics, casual callers, people collecting prescriptions and before home visits. (Verbal reminders or 'reminder' cards on each desk may be required.)
■ Check existing knowledge of people with diabetes with doctors, nurses, administration staff.
■ Check existing registers.

- Check prescription lists.
- Check existing 'labelled diabetes' patient records.
- Check patients new to the practice.
- Note those newly diagnosed (from hospital, surgery or home screening visits).
- Be extra vigilant for people treated with diet alone.
- Check records of regular home visits (for housebound).
- Posters in surgery (Fig. 5.3).
- Maintain communication about diabetes with all members of the primary care team, especially those caring for elderly people and people with mental illness/learning disability.
- Make contact with the local pharmacist(s) who may also have a list or knowledge of the local diabetes population.
- Include any branch surgery population for total practice numbers identified.

Fig. 5.3 Identification poster for surgery use

Do you have diabetes?

Are you treated with:

- **Diet?**
- **Tablets?**
- **Insulin?**

**For your care,
please make sure
we know.**

Thank you

To find out whether the practice has the expected prevalence (number of people with known diabetes), it is necessary to know:

- The total population covered by the practice (total list size).
- Percentage of elderly people (i.e. those over 65 years of age) in the practice population.
- Ethnic composition of the practice population.

A practice with a total list size of 2,200 people with a mainly white population and an average number aged 65 years or over would expect to have at least 1.5–2% (33–44 people) identified with diabetes. About five of these might be type 1 diabetes and the remainder type 2 diabetes (treated with diet, diet and tablets, or diet and insulin).

Once identified, the name should be added to the list and the patient records labelled 'diabetes'. The list of names forms the basis of a 'diabetes' register (on computer or handwritten).

The practice diabetes register

It is required by the Health Authority that registers of people with diabetes are provided by practices that are in CDM payments. District-wide registers are also developing. Requirements for these may be discussed and local guidelines should be followed. A register is needed for the following reasons.

- To *know* how many people have diabetes in the practice.
- To *ensure* that care is available and provided for all people with diabetes in the practice.
- To *control* care provision, i.e. by the primary care team, hospital-based team, if shared, or where care is inadequate.
- To *highlight* care provision that may be inadequate in treatment, education, support and surveillance. For example, where health care is provided by those with no special interest in diabetes, or where the person with diabetes may not be in permanent residence, e.g. students, businessmen, travellers, ethnic minority groups unaware of health care. People with diabetes treated with diet alone may also receive inadequate care.
- To *achieve the aim of organised individualised care* by knowing:
  - the population with diabetes
  - where care is provided (and by whom)
  - what care is provided
  - the standard of care provision.

The register is invaluable in the 'tracking' of people with diabetes who fail to attend or do not attend hospital or general practice for their care, or who may be 'lost' between the two.

Setting up the register

1. Collect the list of names of people identified with diabetes.
2. Take out records – make a list of names (include those at branch surgeries).

3. Note the following:
   (a) Name (address if required)
   (b) Date of birth
   (c) Duration of diabetes (not always possible)
   (d) Treatment – diet, diet and tablets, or diet and insulin
   (e) Identified complications of diabetes (or important associated medical problems):
      (i) retinopathy
      (ii) neuropathy (peripheral/autonomic)
      (iii) nephropathy
      (iv) cardiovascular disease
      (v) peripheral vascular disease
      (this information will be available from hospital letters after clinic appointments)
   (f) Where care is provided, e.g. specialist diabetes physician, other hospital physician, general practitioner, both or none. (The information regarding specialist/other physicians is obtained by checking the letter heading and knowing who the specialist physicians are in the district.)

Figure 5.4 shows an example of a diabetes register.

Maintaining a diabetes register

- A named person in the practice should take responsibility for maintaining the register.
- Any changes (additions, deletions, demographic, treatment, complications or care provision) should be noted as they occur.
- Training is required for a new person taking on this responsibility.
- The system devised for the maintenance of the register should be as simple as possible.
- The register will form the basis of the follow-up and recall system for diabetes care in the practice.

Links with specialist services

Before setting up the practice diabetes service, it is important to know where appropriate referrals to specialist services will be made, what diabetes services are available and the best way of obtaining them.

Contact with the appropriate diabetes team should provide the following necessary information:

Fig. 5.4 Sample diabetes register

Diabetes Register									
Name	Date of Birth	On Diet	On Tablets	On Insulin	Any Problems/Complications	Consultant Initials Hospital	Where Seen GP	Where Seen Both	
1									
2									
3									
4									
5									
6									
7									
8									
9									
10									

- The name(s) of the local diabetes physician(s) (diabetologists).
- Names of diabetes nurse specialists.
- Details of hospital diabetes clinics (where and when clinics are held) including collaborative clinics, e.g. for foot, renal and antenatal care.
- Name(s) of paediatrician(s) with an interest in diabetes.
- Diabetes nurse specialist caring for children (may be separate or part of the diabetes nurse team).
- Details of diabetes clinics for children including collaborative clinics, e.g. for teenagers, young people.
- Details of any district diabetes services provided for elderly people.
- Details of availability and access to diabetes centres – by people with diabetes and by the practice team.
- Advice, information and materials that may be identified as needed by the practice before setting up the service.
- Information regarding self-help groups for people with diabetes, e.g. local branches of Diabetes UK – for adults and/or parents/children.
- Contact for the national charity Diabetes UK.

Links with dietetic services

Obtain information on the following:

- What district information is available regarding dietetic advice?
- Who provides dietetic advice in the district?
- What dietetic advice is provided for people with diabetes seen in the general practice setting?
- Where and when are dietetic sessions available for people with diabetes, who have been referred by the general practitioner?

Links with chiropody (podiatry) services

Obtain information on the following:

- What district information is available regarding feet and shoe care?
- Who provides chiropody/podiatry services in the district?
- Where and when are chiropody/podiatry services available local to the practice (or perhaps they may be organised in the practice, either already for the practice population, or can people with diabetes be added in to an existing practice chiropody/podiatry service)?
- Who and where are private chiropodists/podiatrists (state registered) providing a service local to the practice?

Fig. 5.5 Advertising the practice diabetes service

Diabetes care

A new service for people with diabetes

- **To provide treatment, information and regular checks (if not provided elsewhere)**

- **Held in this surgery**

- **Every Wednesday morning starting at 10.30 am (other times will be arranged if required)**

- **Takes about 20 minutes**

- **Appointment times given**

- **Please ask at reception for details**

Links with other agencies

It may also be helpful to have available information on the following:

- Local support groups (for many general health problems, e.g. stroke support groups, Alcoholics Anonymous – addresses available from local or central libraries).
- Prescription exemption; Disabled living allowance.
- Opticians/optometrists (local diabetes retinal screening services).
- Shoe-fitting services.
- Health food shops (in case this advice is requested).
- Dentists.
- Care and after care services (for walking sticks, frames, commodes, continence supplies, etc.).

Fig. 5.6 Example of a standard letter

Practice Telephone No: 222333
The Medical Practice
Woolly End Road
Airedale Edge
SHEFFIELD
South Yorkshire S2 3AS

January 2001

Mrs P Johnson
The Tannery
Black Terrace
SHEFFIELD S1 1XX

Dear Mrs Johnson

We will shortly be starting a new service of health care for people with diabetes attending the practice. The service will include a review of treatment, information and regular checks.

The service will be provided in the practice (address above) every Wednesday morning, starting at 10.30 am (other times will be arranged if required). The appointment should only take about 20 minutes.

We have made an appointment for you to attend on Wednesday 18 April 2001 at 11 am. Should this time not be convenient, perhaps you could let us know (telephone number at top of letter) and we will arrange another time.

Please bring with you any written food plan (diet sheet) you have been following, your record of urine or blood tests (if you keep a record) and a fresh urine sample.

We look forward to seeing you.

Yours sincerely

Dr A Smith   Mrs M Jones
General Practitioner   Practice Nurse

Advertising the practice diabetes service

Once the people with diabetes are identified and the service planned, notice of this needs to be given. This can be done (1) by posters targeting anyone attending the practice for health care (Fig. 5.5) or (2) by letter to individuals inviting them to attend for diabetes care (Fig. 5.6).

Further reading

Diabetes UK (2000). *New Diagnostic Criteria for Diabetes: summary of changes*. Factsheet. London: Diabetes UK.

Report of the Expert Committee on the Diagnosis and Classification of Diabetes Mellitus (1997). *Diabetes Care* **20**: 1183–97.

Shaw KM, Cummings MH (1997). Revised recommendations for diabetes diagnosis and classification. *Practical Diabetes International* **14**: 121.

Providing the service

Example of locally agreed guidelines for clinical management
Example of criteria for hospital referral
Sample protocol for performing a routine review
Sample protocol for performing an annual review
Recall and follow-up

Example of locally agreed guidelines for clinical management

(This is based on *Recommendations for the Management of Diabetes in Primary Care 1993*, British Diabetic Association.)

Suggested protocol for initial assessment of newly diagnosed patients

1. A patient who is ill, where ketonuria is present or blood glucose is greater than 25 mmol/l, requires hospital referral within 24 hours.
2. Patients under 30 years of age, pregnant women and all those diagnosed with type 1 diabetes should be referred to diabetes centres/services for initial treatment and education.
3. Children presenting with glycosuria should be referred to appropriate paediatric units.
4. The protocol (items 1–17) should be carried out over several visits during a period of about 12 weeks. Baseline measurements for annual review will be available at the end of this time.
5. Specific education and information about diabetes and self-management are not included in the following protocols (see Chapter 14).

Protocol

1. Enter patient details on practice diabetes register.

2. Discuss general aspects of diabetes, enquire about any family history and history of illness leading to diagnosis.
3. Listen and respond to preconceived ideas and anxieties. Establish existing knowledge of diabetes.
4. Discuss general health.
5. Weigh patient and measure height. Calculate body mass index (BMI) and agree target for ideal body weight.

$$BMI = Weight\ in\ kilograms/(Height\ in\ metres)^2$$

6. Test urine for glucose, ketones and protein.
7. Measure blood pressure.
8. Test blood for glucose, renal function, HbA1c.
9. Consider measuring random or fasting cholesterol and triglyceride levels in people under 65 years. Ideally, these should be measured after a period of treatment because initial high triglycerides will fall to normal levels when blood glucose levels are better controlled.
10. Practices should carry out the following tests on diagnosis and annually if necessary:
    - Full blood count
    - ECG
    - Microalbumin
    - Liver function tests
    - Blood glucose
    - Thyroid function tests.
11. Give simple explanation of diabetes, and discuss any fears that the patient may have.
12. Discuss lifestyle in relation to diabetes; record drinking and smoking, advise strongly against the latter.
13. Examine for complications of diabetes:
    - Lower limbs
    - Peripheral pulses and sensation
    - Refer to local diabetes retinal screening services
    - Mid-stream urine (MSU) – if appropriate.
14. Discuss food, meal planning and initiate advice regarding eating plan (Figs 6.1 and 6.2).
15. Record information in the practice records and in diabetes cooperation cards, if used.
16. Arrange prescription (if required) and next appointment – regular and early reviews will be necessary until the patient has a good understanding of diabetes and metabolic control is achieved.

Fig. 6.1 A scheme for managing people with type 2 diabetes – the overweight (BMI > 27)

Fig. 6.1

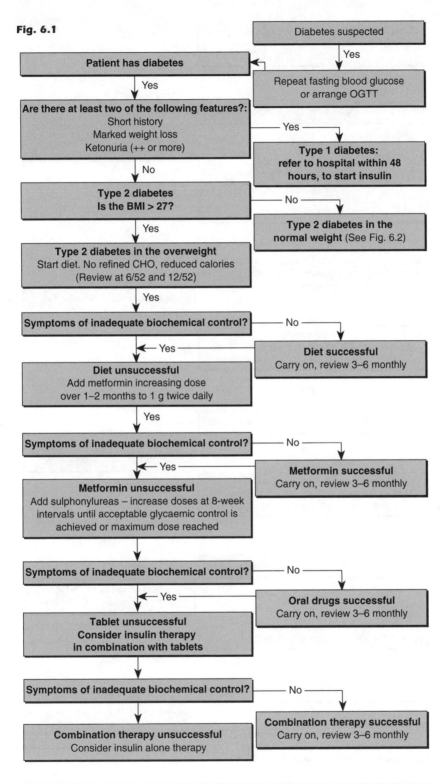

Diabetes suspected

↓ Yes

Repeat fasting blood glucose
or arrange OGTT

Patient has diabetes

↓ Yes

Are there at least two of the following features?:
Short history
Marked weight loss
Ketonuria (++ or more)

— Yes —

Type 1 diabetes:
refer to hospital within 48
hours, to start insulin

↓ No

Type 2 diabetes
Is the BMI > 27?

— No —

Type 2 diabetes in the
normal weight (See Fig. 6.2)

↓ Yes

Type 2 diabetes in the overweight
Start diet. No refined CHO, reduced calories
(Review at 6/52 and 12/52)

↓ Yes

Symptoms of inadequate biochemical control? — No —

Diet successful
Carry on, review 3–6 monthly

← Yes —

Diet unsuccessful
Add metformin increasing dose
over 1–2 months to 1 g twice daily

↓ Yes

Symptoms of inadequate biochemical control? — No —

Metformin successful
Carry on, review 3–6 monthly

← Yes —

Metformin unsuccessful
Add sulphonylureas – increase doses at 8-week
intervals until acceptable glycaemic control is
achieved or maximum dose reached

↓

Symptoms of inadequate biochemical control? — No —

Oral drugs successful
Carry on, review 3–6 monthly

← Yes —

Tablet unsuccessful
Consider insulin therapy
in combination with tablets

↓

Symptoms of inadequate biochemical control? — No —

Combination therapy successful
Carry on, review 3–6 monthly

↓

Combination therapy unsuccessful
Consider insulin alone therapy

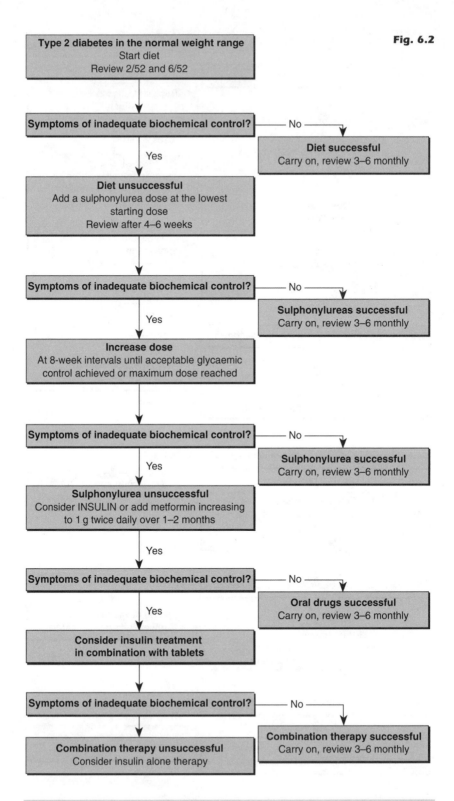

Fig. 6.2

Type 2 diabetes in the normal weight range
Start diet
Review 2/52 and 6/52

Symptoms of inadequate biochemical control? —— No ——

Diet successful
Carry on, review 3–6 monthly

Yes

Diet unsuccessful
Add a sulphonylurea dose at the lowest
starting dose
Review after 4–6 weeks

Symptoms of inadequate biochemical control? —— No ——

Sulphonylureas successful
Carry on, review 3–6 monthly

Yes

Increase dose
At 8-week intervals until acceptable glycaemic
control achieved or maximum dose reached

Symptoms of inadequate biochemical control? —— No ——

Sulphonylurea successful
Carry on, review 3–6 monthly

Yes

Sulphonylurea unsuccessful
Consider INSULIN or add metformin increasing
to 1 g twice daily over 1–2 months

Yes

Symptoms of inadequate biochemical control? —— No ——

Oral drugs successful
Carry on, review 3–6 monthly

Yes

**Consider insulin treatment
in combination with tablets**

Symptoms of inadequate biochemical control? —— No ——

Combination therapy successful
Carry on, review 3–6 monthly

Combination therapy unsuccessful
Consider insulin alone therapy

Fig. 6.2 A scheme for managing type 2 diabetes – the normal weight

17. Notify information to district diabetes register.
18. It is important to note that patients must be informed if data are held on a register outside the practice.

Example of criteria for hospital referral

Referral is required in the following situations.

Urgent (telephone referral within 24 hours)

- For protracted vomiting – an emergency referral is required.
- For moderate or heavy ketonuria.
- For an acutely infected or ischaemic foot.
- In the newly diagnosed (type 1 diabetes).
- If insulin is needed (type 2 diabetes).
- For an unplanned pregnancy.

Routine

- If a pregnancy is planned.
- If insulin treatment is required (referral should be urgent in the newly diagnosed).
- Problems in patient management, e.g. if targets for control are not being met.
- If complications are detected, for example:
  - persistent proteinuria
  - raised serum creatinine
  - retinopathy
  - unexplained loss of vision
  - painful neuropathy, mononeuropathy, amyotrophy
  - deteriorating condition of feet
  - uncontrolled hypertension
  - impotence.
- Psychological problems complicating diabetes, for example:
  - failure to accept diagnosis
  - morbid fear of complications
  - family difficulties.

Sample protocol for performing a routine review

Ensure that patients with established diabetes are included on the diabetes register and are booked for regular appointments. A system for identifying and recalling defaulters should be organised and a policy agreed for the frequency of follow-up of people with diabetes. For routine visits where management and understanding of the condition are established and uncomplicated, these may be required only two or three times a year.

Protocol

1. Weigh patient (keep weight confidential, i.e. between patient and health care professional).
2. Test urine for glucose, ketones and protein; check MSU if protein present.
3. Take blood sample for HbA1c (preferably take this sample [and any other blood samples] 7–10 days before review appointment so that results are available for discussion with patient).
4. Discuss the patient's general progress and well-being, enquire about any problems (life changes, diet, etc.). If treatment with insulin – check injection sites.
5. Identify and discuss any weak spots in knowledge of diabetes and self-management skills.
6. Perform examinations or investigations as required (preferably 7–10 days before review appointment).
7. Discuss and agree targets with the patient – see guidelines in Table 6.1.
8. Record all details in diabetes record card and/or practice record.
9. Arrange next appointment.

Sample protocol for performing an annual review

Protocol

1. Weigh patient.
2. Urinalysis: glucose/albumin/ketones.
   Arrange MSU if protein/blood present.
   Screen for microalbuminuria (see box on pages 82–3).

Table 6.1 A guide to glycaemic control – targets

Biochemical indices of glycaemic control	Age (years)		
	30–50	**50–70**	**>70**
Fasting blood glucose < 8 mmol/l HbA1c < 9%	Good	Depends upon their general medical health	May be over control/at high risk of hypoglycaemia on sulphonylureas/ insulin
Fasting blood glucose 8–11 mmol/l HbA1c > 9–10.5%	Undesirable but sometimes inevitable		Acceptable
Fasting blood glucose > 11 mmol/l HbA1c > 11%	Undesirable	Undesirable	Undesirable but sometimes inevitable

3. Enquire about:
   - subjective changes in eyes and feet
   - claudication
   - neuropathy symptoms, impotence
   - chest pain, shortness of breath.
4. Examine for diabetic complications:
   - blood pressure
   - peripheral pulses and sensation
   - lower limbs
   - visual acuity
   - fundoscopy with dilated pupils
   - arrange MSU, if appropriate.
5. Take blood sample for:
   - blood glucose (feed back result)
   - HbA1c (performed in advance of annual review)
   - creatinine
   - cholesterol – this is recommended for those under 65 years of age, if found to be high at previous testing (these tests should be performed in advance of the annual review).

Screening for microalbuminuria

There is now sufficient evidence to recommend screening for microalbuminuria in selected groups of people with diabetes. Microalbuminuria is the excretion of traces of protein in the urine in amounts undetectable using dipsticks, as an indicator of early, possibly treatable, renal disease.

Type 1 diabetes
People with type 1 diabetes run a 30–40% chance of developing diabetic nephropathy in their lifetime, and also other complications. The time when they are most likely to develop nephropathy is after between 10 and 25 years of diabetes. Those who develop microalbuminuria between 5 and 15 years after diagnosis of the condition have about an 80% chance of progressing to renal failure in 10 years. Those who have not developed albuminuria after 30 years of diabetes are less likely to progress to renal failure.

Overt proteinuria is preceded by 2–5 years of increasing quantities of protein excretion and it is this that can be detected by specialised microalbuminuria testing strips. The healthy, non-diabetic person excretes 10 mg/day of albumin, and this can be detected by Albustix at concentrations of 0.5 g/l or 300 mg/day or over. Microalbuminuria refers to levels of 20–200 mg/day.

Type 2 diabetes
Microalbuminuria in people with type 2 diabetes does not have the same predictive value as it does in type 1 diabetes, because many of these people have macrovascular disease at diagnosis of type 2 diabetes and there is no clear link between microalbuminuria and renal disease in these cases. It seems appropriate therefore not to screen for microalbuminuria in these people, but to concentrate on blood glucose and blood pressure control.

Hypertension
It is known that careful antihypertensive treatment in patients with overt nephropathy can slow down the deterioration in renal function. Treatment is most effective in those whose levels of creatinine have already begun to rise. ACE inhibitors have been shown to be most effective in this situation (lowering the BP to 140/80 or less).

Who should be screened?
On current evidence, it seems reasonable to screen people who have had type 1 diabetes for between 5 and 15 years.

Method of screening
This would be carried out mainly in hospitals. First, patients are asked to bring in an early morning urine sample and the albumin/creatinine ratio is measured (normal values are 2.5 mg/mol for men and 4.5 mg/mol for women); then, in those who screen positive, an MSU should be taken. If infection is excluded, two timed urine specimens are done (between 22:00 and 08:00). Results are averaged and any rates over 30 μg/min are significant. Annual screening is recommended. It should be noted that the sticks are expensive and have a short shelf-life.

Action on positive results
For those people who test positive and have hypertension, an ACE inhibitor should be used to lower the BP to <140/90. This treatment could also be considered for those who have normotension.

This screening information has been produced with permission from material written by Dr Simon Heller (Consultant Physician) and consolidated by Dr Jenny Stephenson (General Practitioner).

6. Discuss the patient's general progress and well-being, enquire about any problems relating to diabetes and whether any supplies are needed. If treatment with insulin – check injection sites.
7. Record information in the records and cooperation card if used.
8. Arrange prescription (if required) and next appointment.
9. Notify information to the district diabetes register.

Recall and follow-up

People with diabetes (whether patients new to the practice or newly diagnosed) need to understand how the diabetes service is organised; the system of recall and follow-up should be explained. Should an individual have a problem regarding attendance (caused by employment shifts or family commitments), it is important that these problems are identified early on. The practice diabetes service should be sufficiently flexible to accommodate certain particular difficulties and incorporate visits for surveillance to the housebound receiving no other health care.

Where no system is in existence, the following procedure is recommended:

1. Note telephone number on records.

2. Use a standard letter (see Fig. 5.6 in Chapter 5) inviting new patients to attend.
3. Agree a follow-up appointment at the end of each visit.
4. Fill in an appointment card with the agreed date and time and give it to the patient before his or her departure.
5. Use a clinic diary (or card index system). Fill this in with the agreed times for each follow-up visit to avoid over- or under-booking (a computer system may be useful here).
6. Allow enough time for each patient: 20 minutes for a routine follow-up visit, 30 minutes for an initial visit or an annual review.
7. Allow 5 minutes between each patient and 15 minutes (or more) at the end of each session for recording information and dealing with follow-up work (such as organising dietitian, referral letters, chiropody/podiatry).
8. Allow for a little leeway in each session if possible, for a person with diabetes requesting an unexpected or urgent visit.

Frequency of recall and follow-up

Note: it is not necessary for people with diabetes to attend the practice every week/month for the checking of blood glucose levels (except in unusual circumstances). A scheme such as this provides no benefit, promotes diabetes as an illness and discourages self-management.

Frequency of recall and follow-up may depend on the following:

■ Age, state and needs of the patient; these may relate to:
   ◆ being newly diagnosed
   ◆ being new to the practice
   ◆ being discharged from hospital care
   ◆ requirement for help with losing weight
   ◆ feet at risk
   ◆ impaired vision
   ◆ mobility
   ◆ glycaemic control
   ◆ other medical problems (which may affect diabetes)
   ◆ education requirements
   ◆ support (emotional) (family/other problems).
■ Realistic recall targets relating to numbers to be seen in the practice cared for by practice team only and those receiving shared care.
■ Frequency of hospital appointments where care is shared.
■ Available transport.

Table 6.2 An example of a practice annual recall system

Sample
Practice Register, Recall And Follow Up
Year

Name	Date of birth	Jan	Feb	Mar	April	May	June	July	Aug	Sept	Oct	Nov	Dec	Foot check	Eye check	Home visit	New patient	New diagnosis	IDDM NIDDM both	H GP
1 Elsie Brown	10.2.20	C X		C FTA	✓									✓			✓		NI	GP
2																			NI	GP
3 John White	12.10.32		C X / C X / C X	C / ✓ / ✓										✓	✓			✓	NI	GP
4															✓	✓				
5 Freda Green	21.9.12				C X						NB FLU ✓			✓	✓	✓			NI	GP
6						C X / H					✓			✓	✓					
7 Martin Block	15.6.80		C X / H															✓	–	H child
8																				
9																				
10																				

Key	✓ Due	C ✓ Called	C X Seen	FTA Failed to attend

- Doctor/nurse time allocated/available.
- Time of year relating to practice workload/annual leave by key team members.

In a small practice, diabetes sessions may only be required monthly or even bi-monthly. A larger practice or a practice with a large number of people with diabetes (e.g. where there is a high ethnic composition) may require weekly sessions.

Specific sessions may be allocated for the annual review, or perhaps for visual acuity testing followed by fundoscopy where extra time may be required. Alternatively these may be carried out at the appropriate time in the year (at the same time each year) at a routine session.

The number of appointments for diabetes sessions or surgery visits *should not be excessive if sufficient time has been spent on clinical care and education.* Urgent or costly treatment may be avoided for the same reason:

- Every person with diabetes should be seen at least twice a year (every 6 months).
- People newly diagnosed or those experiencing problems may need weekly visits for a while, to incorporate baseline measurements and minimum education requirements.

Notes
- Elderly people with diabetes, sometimes with complications and/or multiple medical problems, should be reviewed periodically in relation to visits to the practice, hospital or for other health care.
- It is important to ensure that time, cost and travel are not proving too great a burden and are truly beneficial to each person concerned.
- The recall and follow-up system should be flexible and responsive to the needs of each patient, reflecting organised, individualised care.

References

Diabetes UK (2000). *New Diagnostic Criteria for Diabetes: summary of changes*. Factsheet. London: Diabetes UK.

Heller SR (1993). *Guidelines for Clinical Management*. Diabetes Care in Sheffield FHSA Working Party/Diabetologists.

UKPDS 33. *Lancet* 1998; **352**: 837–53.

UKPDS 34. *Lancet* 1998; **352**: 854–65.

UKPDS 35. *BMJ* 2000; **321**: 405–12.

UKPDS 36. *BMJ* 2000; **321**: 412–19.

UKPDS 38. *BMJ* 1998; **317**: 703–13.

UKPDS 39. *BMJ* 1998; **317**: 713–20.

7 Treating diabetes

Aims of treatment

- To relieve symptoms.
- To ensure a satisfactory lifestyle.
- To prevent unwanted effects of treatment (i.e. hypoglycaemia, side effects of drugs).
- To reduce the risks of acute complications (hypoglycaemia, hyperglycaemia).
- To reduce the risks of long-term complications

Relieving symptoms

Treatment should aim first of all to relieve symptoms. Assessment of symptoms should come before assessment of blood glucose control. Symptoms will decrease as blood glucose levels fall (these levels varying from person to person). People with diabetes soon learn the association between symptoms and hyperglycaemia and the benefits of treatment in renewed energy and an improved sense of well-being.

Ensuring a satisfactory lifestyle

People with diabetes and their families need sufficient information to make any lifestyle adjustments required by their treatment and monitoring, and to enable independence in their management of the condition. It is important that activity, exercise, eating habits, family and social life, and work are all considered in relation to suggested treatment.

Preventing unwanted effects of treatment (hypoglycaemia, side effects of drugs)

Information should be given to the person with diabetes (relative or carer) regarding the effects of treatment, in particular the hypoglycaemic effects of oral hypoglycaemic agents. Information is required on the importance of:

- Regular eating.
- Sufficient consumption of carbohydrate.
- Monitoring of weight (by the person and/or the practice) as a reduction in weight may indicate that a lower drug dose is required.
- Noting and reporting symptoms of hypoglycaemia (see Chapter 9).
- Advice regarding prevention of hypoglycaemia (see Chapters 8 and 9).
- Side effects of drugs prescribed (symptoms and that these should be reported to the care team).

Strategy of treatment for preventing and reducing the risk of diabetic complications (types 1 and 2 diabetes)

- Strongly advise adherence to diet and medication, cessation of smoking, exercise and weight reduction. Stress role of the dietitian, chiropodist (podiatrist) and diabetes care nurses. Ensure diabetes education and advise Diabetes UK membership. Regular follow-up with comprehensive annual review is essential. Twenty per cent of patients with diabetes and early severe complications will be persistent diabetes clinic non-attenders.
- Screening for and effective management of early complications to reduce morbidity and mortality: hypertension, dyslipidaemia, foot ulceration, retinopathy (digital retinal camera) and nephropathy. If neuropathic or ischaemic foot is present, immediate referral to chiropody (podiatry) service is essential.
- Glycaemic control: aim for HbA1c < 7%. Where realistic use metformin early in type 2 diabetes (in overweight patients), because insulin resistance is usually present. Metformin can also be used with insulin in type 2 patients, both as an insulin-sparing manoeuvre, and to improve insulin resistance, reduce hypertension and improve lipid profile. Thiazolidinediones (rosiglitazone and pioglitazone) are now licensed for use in combination with metformin alone or a high-dose sulphonylurea

alone). Use multiple oral agents if needed, e.g. metformin, gliclazide (or tolbutamide) and acarbose. Use insulin early if HbA1c target is not achieved. Multiple (four/day) insulin injections often needed.

■ Meticulous glycaemic control is essential in pregnancy.

■ Author's note: postprandial glucose regulators (PPGRs) are also licensed for use (e.g. repaglinide and nateglanide). Further information on action, dose, contraindications and side effects for oral hypoglycaemic agents can be found in Chapter 8.

■ Aggressive control of any hypertension > 140/80 mmHg. If secondary complications present, particularly nephropathy, aim for BP < 130/80. Use angiotensin-converting enzyme (ACE) inhibitors as first-line, then diuretics (indapamide 1.5 mg once daily has fewer side effects of hypokalaemia, hyperglycaemia and dyslipidaemia), α blockade with doxazosin, Ca^{2+} channel blockade with a long-acting agent, angiotensin II receptor antagonists or central-acting agents. Assess dietary salt intake.

■ Aspirin 75 mg once daily: Diabetes UK now advocates considering aspirin prophylaxis against cardiovascular events in all patients with diabetes (> 30 years) with any of the following: myocardial infarction, angina, hypertension, diabetic retinopathy, peripheral vascular disease and microalbuminuria. This simple measure is grossly under-implemented. Full guidelines and contraindications can be found in Chapter 8.

■ ACE inhibitors have a special role in preventing diabetic complications. The best data in type 1 patients with proteinuria (500 mg/24 h) are with captopril 50 mg three times daily. In all other groups, lisinopril has a nephropathy licence for the treatment of hypertension in type 2 diabetes with microalbuminuria and normotensive patients with type 1 diabetes. Diabetic retinopathy progression is also significantly slowed by lisinopril in type 1 diabetes.

■ Post-myocardial infarction, most patients will need aspirin, ACE inhibitors and β blockade. β Blockade with atenolol or metoprolol is actually more beneficial to a patient with diabetes than to one without. Lisinoprol and ramipril have proved to be particularly effective in post-myocardial infarction in a patient with diabetes.

■ All patients with myocardial infarction and unstable angina should be considered for statin treatment. Best evidence: cholesterol level 4–7 mmol/l will benefit from pravastatin 40 mg at night. Simvastatin 20–40 mg at night will benefit those with a cholesterol of 5.5–8.0 mmol/l. Exact statin prescribed will depend on local guidelines.

This text for this strategy is taken from Patel (2001) with permission.

Over-treatment and under-treatment should be avoided. Information should be provided regarding the following in relation to treatment prescribed.

Hypoglycaemia (for details see Chapters 8 and 9)
- Symptoms
- Treatment
- Prevention.

Hyperglycaemia (for details see Chapter 9)
- Symptoms
- Treatment
- Prevention.

Reducing the risks of long-term complications

Risks to life and health in diabetes are caused by the following:

- Recognised complications of diabetes
- Cardiovascular disease leading to premature death.

Minimising the risks of complications should include other factors as well as control of blood glucose levels:

- No smoking
- Maintenance of a normal blood pressure
- Good blood glucose control
- Control of serum lipids.

To achieve these, the following are necessary:

- Regular medical examinations
- Support, education and advice in relation to treatment
- Individually negotiated targets for treatment and control
- Targets appropriate to age and ability to achieve them
- Regular assessment of symptoms and well-being.

SUMMARY

1. Treatment must aim to alleviate symptoms and maintain the safety of the person concerned.
2. Simple risk factors should be reduced or eliminated.
3. Targets for control should be individualised and negotiated.
4. Sufficient information should be given to the person with diabetes (relative or carer) to understand their diabetes and achieve independence in its management.

Starting treatment (type 2 diabetes)

Some important points

■ Assess preconceived ideas and knowledge about diabetes and treatment. Reassurance, support and information are needed. People with diabetes, newly diagnosed, are often concerned that they will be on a 'strict diet' for the rest of their lives or frightened that they will be 'on the needle'.

■ Explain that there are three types of treatment of diabetes:
  ◆ modification of food intake (dietary habits)
  ◆ modification of food intake and drugs
  ◆ modification of food intake and insulin.

■ Explain that treatment is ongoing and that it may be changed if symptoms persist and blood glucose levels remain high.

■ Emphasise that, should a change in treatment become necessary, this does not mean failure on the part of the person with diabetes.

■ Explain that the treatment is individually prescribed and that the treatment and its effects are particular to each person.

Note that (1) a young person, newly diagnosed with type 1 diabetes, should be referred to the hospital-based team, and (2) a guide to insulin therapy is provided in Chapter 8.

The treatment

■ Treatment prescribed will depend on the age, weight, lifestyle and any other medical conditions of the person concerned (of particular importance in elderly people).

■ **!WARNING!:** Patients should not be started on treatment with drugs before assessment of their weight, dietary habits and advice on modification of their food intake.

■ **!WARNING!:** No treatment should be started before the diagnosis has been confirmed.

■ Modification of food intake and dietary habits are the first lines of treatment in almost all cases.

■ It is important, when planning treatment, to distinguish between people with diabetes who are of normal weight and those who are overweight.

■ It is usually clinically obvious that the person concerned is overweight. However, a body mass index (BMI) of greater than 27 indicates this condition – the formula for calculating the BMI is given in Chapter 6.

Note: examples of treatment schemes are shown in Figs 6.1 and 6.2 in Chapter 6.

Non-drug treatment

Dietary therapy

■ The 'cornerstones' of treatment are modification of food intake and dietary habits. These should be tried for at least 3 months before drug treatment is considered. Dietary advice, if followed, may well relieve the symptoms and improve metabolic control successfully.

■ Ideally, people with type 2 diabetes should see a dietitian for assessment and individual advice.

■ 'Stop-gap' advice, backed up with written information, is acceptable initially.

■ The practice nurse or other designated members of the primary care team can give dietary advice, if appropriately trained.

■ Access to a hospital-based dietitian should be provided if no community dietitian is available or if there is no trained member of the primary care team able to provide dietary advice.

Healthy eating and diabetes

■ Modification of food intake is almost always the first line of treatment.

■ The diet for a person with diabetes is not 'special', it is a healthy way of eating, recommended for everyone.

■ It is important that an adequate and balanced nutritional intake is maintained (particularly in an elderly person, who may have a diminished appetite).

■ It is important to remember the social aspects of meal planning, shopping, cooking and meal time – in relation to family life. If there is a family life change (i.e. retirement, bereavement of a partner), this can have a profound effect on eating habits.

■ 'Healthy eating' for diabetes is of benefit to all family members. Dietary advice should emphasise this point.

■ No 'special' arrangements are required; adaptations to the usual food eaten are all that is needed.

■ Recommendations for healthy eating and diabetes are given in the list suggested in Fig. 7.1. This list could be used in the surgery as a basic guideline or stop-gap advice.

■ A simple guide (Fig. 7.2) to diet and diabetes for a newly diagnosed person provides advice in more detail until a comprehensive assessment and advice can be provided, by either a dietitian or trained practice nurse.

■ Diabetes UK produces booklets *Eating Well with Diabetes* and *Food and Diabetes: how to get it right*. These booklets provide general dietary advice.

■ For advice about complementary therapies and diabetes, see Chapter 13, 'Education for self-management'.

Fig. 7.1 Healthy eating and diabetes

1. Eat regular meals, i.e. breakfast, mid-day and evening. Some people need healthy snacks in between meals to ensure blood glucose levels do not fall too low.

2. Eat starchy carbohydrate foods with each meal, e.g. bread, potatoes, oats, cereals, Basmati rice, sweet potato, chapatti, yam, couscous.

3. Cut down on fried and fatty foods, e.g. butter, margarine, oil, cheese, fatty meats and pastries/pies. If you need to use fat choose olive- or rapeseed-based oils/margarines.

4. Aim to eat at least five fruits or vegetables each day, e.g. apples, oranges, bananas that are not too ripe, any vegetables you like.

5. Aim to reduce your sugar intake. Cut down on sugar, cakes, confectionery and sugar in drinks. If you need some sweetness in drinks have sweeteners. You can also choose diet pop, no added sugar squash, which taste sweet but have no sugar.

6. Check if you need to lose weight. Choose a realistic target and lose weight slowly (1–2 lb per week or 0.5–1 kg per week).

7. Be careful not to add too much salt in cooking and at the table. Give yourself time to get used to the taste of less salt.

8. Be careful not to drink too much alcohol. Never drink on an empty stomach.

9. Avoid foods labelled 'DIABETIC'. They are expensive and do not help you control your diabetes.

Fig. 7.2 Towards healthy eating

- Eat regularly and do not miss meals. If you get hungry in-between meals then choose healthy snacks such as fresh fruit, vegetable sticks, diet yogurt, two Rich Tea biscuits or a slice of bread.

- Eat starchy carbohydrate foods at each meal, e.g. bread, potatoes, oats, cereals, Basmati rice, sweet potato, chapatti, yam, couscous.

- Avoid sugar and sugary foods. Try to reduce your sweet tooth by having unsweetened drinks. If you really need some sweetness use a sweetener (Canderel, Sweetex, supermarkets' own brands). Choose diet/no added sugar drinks and reduced sugar products, e.g. reduced sugar jam/ marmalade, sugar-free desserts, sugar-free jelly. Avoid sweets, biscuits, cakes and all foods labelled 'DIABETIC'.

- Eat less fat. Use semi-skimmed/skimmed milk and margarines labelled 'low-fat spread'. Choose lean meats and cut away all visible fat. Try to grill, bake, steam or cook with very little olive/rapeseed oil. Cut down on fatty foods such as chips, cheese, pastries and pies. Look for foods labelled 'low/reduced fat', but make sure that they are also low in sugar too.

Dietary recommendations for people with diabetes

A combination of up-to-date research and the Diabetes UK's dietary recommendations for people with diabetes has seen many changes in the advice. These can be summarised as follows.

Energy

- Keep energy intake fairly constant (weight variation is an indicator of this).
- Fluctuations of energy intake may have an effect on blood glucose levels.
- Eat regularly.
- Foods high in energy, such as fatty meat, fried foods, dairy products, and sugary foods and drinks, can cause deterioration in blood glucose control.

Carbohydrate

- At least half of the energy intake should come from starchy carbohydrate foods such as bread, potatoes, Basmati rice, pasta, cereals, yam, sweet potato, chapatti and pitta bread.
- The concept of glycaemic index (see page 99) has allowed more flexibility in dietary intake and shows that certain types of starchy carbohydrate foods help control blood glucose levels more effectively.
- Rapidly absorbed carbohydrate foods (e.g. sweets, chocolates, sweet drinks) should be kept for special occasions and situations such as illness, or as a snack before strenuous activity.
- Hypos should be treated with rapidly absorbed carbohydrate, e.g. glucose tablets, ordinary fizzy drinks, ordinary Lucozade or glucose drinks. Hypos should not be treated with chocolate, cakes or biscuits. These do not allow a quick enough increase in blood glucose levels to help hypos.
- Fibre has proved not to be as beneficial in controlling blood glucose levels as was once thought. Only 'soluble fibre' helps control blood glucose levels, e.g. pulses, oats, pasta, fruit and vegetables. Having insoluble fibre in 'wholemeal' versions does not actually help control blood glucose levels any more than the 'white' versions. However, fibre does have other health benefits, such as reducing the risk of bowel cancer, diverticular disease and constipation. Plenty of fluids are needed to help this type of fibre to work properly.
- Foods lower in energy content than their sweetened equivalents, such as low-calorie squashes, diet fizzy drinks, diet yoghurts, fruit tinned in natural juice and artificial sweeteners, may be used.
- Food on your plate is a useful tool for menu planning (Fig. 7.3). You can enlarge this figure by photocopying and give it to your patients.

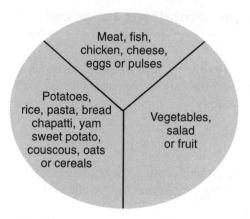

Fig. 7.3 Food on your plate (original plate model designed by Ruth Webber, modified by Surinder Ghatoray). Balance your meals with a 'Y' on your plate. Make sure you drink plenty with your meals and in between meals also.

■ Portion sizes recommended need to be adjusted according to weight, but the balance is still the same.

Fat

■ Monounsaturated fats should be used if they are needed in cooking. These have the added benefit of lowering fasting plasma triglyceride and VLDL-cholesterol concentrations, and increasing HDL-cholesterol with no changes in LDL-cholesterol. Monounsaturated fats include olive oil and pure vegetable oil made from rapeseed.
■ Eat less fatty meat and meat products; choose smaller portions of meat, fish and poultry.
■ Cut down on high-fat diary products, such as cheese, butter and cream.
■ Use a low-fat spread instead of butter or margarine.
■ Use skimmed or semi-skimmed milk instead of whole milk. Skimmed milk has fewer calories but some people find that semi-skimmed milk is more palatable initially when changing from full-fat milk.

Salt

Reduce salt intake by:

■ Eating fewer salty foods, such as pre-cooked meats, smoked fish or cheese.
■ Add less salt during cooking.
■ Cut down on salt added at the table.

Alcohol

■ A maximum of three 'units' for men and two for women per day is recommended, after consultation with a physician.

■ 1 'unit' = half pint of ordinary beer or lager = a single measure of spirits (whisky, gin, rum, vodka, etc.) = a glass of wine = a measure of vermouth or aperitif.

■ It is better to drink less alcohol. If weight is a problem, consumption should be limited to one drink per day.

■ Aim to have at least two to three alcohol-free days each week.

■ Low-carbohydrate beers and lagers should be avoided. These are high in calories and alcohol.

■ High-alcohol beers, special brews and 'Pils'-type alcohol should be avoided. Just stick to ordinary beers and lagers, and spirits with a low sugar content.

■ Alcohol lowers the blood sugar, so it is important not to drink on an empty stomach. Meals or snacks should not be replaced with alcohol.

Special diabetic foods

■ These are not recommended. They may contain more fat or energy than other foods and may be low in fibre.

■ Sorbitol is used to sweeten them and this may cause diarrhoea.

■ Fructose may also be used in diabetic products. This has the same energy value as sugar. No more than 25 g/day should be taken.

■ A small piece of ordinary (sweetened) cake or chocolate on the odd occasion, preferably taken at the end of a meal, is not likely to be harmful. Remember that these foods may put weight on if eaten too often.

■ Diabetic squashes are no better than low-calorie squashes found in most supermarkets. Use 'low-calorie', 'diet' or 'sugar-free' drinks.

Important

■ Diabetic foods are expensive and unnecessary

■ Diabetes UK's recommendations regarding the use of sugar: if the person with diabetes is not overweight and follows a high starchy carbohydrate, high-fibre, low-fat diet, up to 25 g of sugar can be used each day. This should be spread throughout the day and used in combination with high-fibre foods where possible. It should not be used in drinks or on cereals where artificial sweeteners can be used.

Note

Further helpful hints, recipes and cooking tips are available from local dietitians and Diabetes UK, including special cultural modifications, e.g. for the south Asian (i.e. from the Indian subcontinent) or African–Caribbean person with diabetes. For more information on the eating patterns and advice to give African–Caribbean people and people from south Asia, see Chapter 12.

Schedule of dietary treatment for people with type 2 diabetes who are overweight

- Assess food and alcohol intake (types of food and alcohol enjoyed and amounts taken during the day).
- Assess activity/exercise taken (on a daily basis).
- Discuss targets for weight loss – short and long term. These targets should be realistic, possible and desired by the person with diabetes.
- Provide appropriate advice.
- Monitor and support regularly, e.g. monthly if weight loss is not seen within 3 months and blood sugar remains elevated.
- Aim for a slow weight loss by reducing your food intake, but make sure that you do not miss meals. Aim to lose half to one kilogram per week or 1 to 2 pounds per week.

Schedule of dietary treatment for people with type 2 diabetes who are of normal weight

- Assess food and alcohol intake (types of foods and alcohol enjoyed and amounts taken during the day).
- Assess activity/exercise taken (on a daily basis).
- Discuss targets for maintaining weight – short and long term.
- Provide appropriate advice.
- Encourage regular activity and exercise.
- Monitor at regular intervals to check on weight regulation and blood sugar control.

Activity for health

- Physical activity will help with weight loss, regulate blood glucose levels and improve insulin sensitivity.
- Advice about exercise should be realistic and possible, and should include information on local facilities available (e.g. swimming, health clubs). It is important to find out what the person with diabetes enjoys doing.

■ Information provided should include costs, which may be prohibitive for some people.
■ Advice regarding exercise (particularly for those not used to it) should be given only in association with a medical examination and advice.
■ Recommendations from the Health Education Authority (1998) state:

> ... for improved health and to help with weight management, adults should try to build up gradually to take half-an-hour of moderate intensity physical activity on five or more days of the week. Activities like brisk walking, cycling, swimming, dancing and gardening are good options.

■ It is important to build any activity levels slowly and ideally the pace should make you breathe a little faster, but not be so out of breath that you can't talk. The 30 min can be spread throughout the day in 5- to 10-min slots.

Glycaemic index

Glycaemic index (GI) is very much in vogue and you may be approached by people with diabetes asking about this very subject. Foods are ranked high (> 70) (glucose, baked potato, cornflakes, digestive biscuits), intermediate (55–70) (Basmati rice, Taco shells, banana) and low (< 55) (apple, plain sponge cake, lentils, Rich Tea biscuits).

Evidence shows that foods with a low GI create a slow rise in blood sugars, leading to better overall control of blood sugars – a benefit to people with diabetes. Other positive aspects of GI are reducing cardiac risk factors, benefits for insulin resistance and reducing the risk of type 2 diabetes. Studies published about GI point to improved glycaemic control. Having a low GI meal actually helps in glycaemic control of the next meal! Eating foods with low GIs can reduce the risk of hypos. It is no longer good practice to advise chocolate when someone has a hypo because the GI of chocolate is not high enough to increase blood sugars quickly enough. Everyone digests foods at different rates, so the GI concept is not the answer for everyone. Home monitoring helps the individual to see if dietary changes make a difference.

The following are examples of low GI foods:

Breakfast cereals: porridge oats, All Bran, unsweetened toasted muesli

Grains, pasta and Basmati rice

Breads: wholegrain breads, rye bread and fruit loaf (white); replace with grains, pasta and rice at times to help reduce the GI and add variety to your meals

Pulses, dhals and beans: use as an alternative to meat or add into dishes

Vegetables: carrots, green peas, sweet corn, boiled sweet potato, yam

Fruits and fruit juices: GI increases as fruit ripens, so eat fresh fruit. Have as a between-meal snack instead of biscuits; ensures the recommended five portions of fruit and vegetables a day. Fruit juices are fine, but not in excess.

Sweet foods: OK to have some foods containing sugar; low GI sweet foods include a small piece plain sponge cake, two Rich Tea (not digestive!) and oatmeal biscuits, six small squares of milk/plain chocolate, and diet yogurt or two scoops of low-fat ice-cream

Snack and convenience foods: fish fingers, peanuts (preferably unsalted), low-fat popcorn, plain crisps (watch the weight!), sausages and pulse-based soups

Further reading

British Diabetic Association Report (1992). Dietary recommendations for people with diabetes. *Diabetic Medicine* **9**: 189–202.

Department of Nutrition and Diabetes (1990). *Community Nutrition Information.* Sheffield Health Authority.

National Service Framework for Coronary Heart Disease (2000). Department of Health, PO Box 777, London SE1 6XH. Tel: NHS Response line – 0870 1555 455; fax: 01623 724524 (email: doh@prolog.uk.com) (Website: www.doh.gov.uk./nsf/coronary.htm)

Patel V (2001). What the NSF will bring. Strategy for the Prevention of Diabetic Complications. *Abstract in Conference Proceedings: Diabetes is a Cardiovascular Disease.* The First Joint Meeting of the Primary Care Cardiovascular Society, Diabetes UK and Health Care Section of the British Hyperlipidaemia Association. International Conference Centre, Birmingham, 28 February 2001.

Research Unit, Royal College of Physicians, British Diabetic Association and Royal College of General Practitioners (1993). *Guidelines for good practice in the diagnosis and treatment of non-insulin-dependent diabetes mellitus.* London: RCP.

Scottish Intercollegiate Guidelines Network (SIGN) (1996). Edinburgh.

Wood D, Durrington, Poulter N, McInnes G, Rees A, Wray (1998) Joint British recommendations on prevention of coronary heart disease in clinical practice. *Heart* **80**(suppl 2). British Cardiac Society. London: BMJ Publishing Group.

Drug and insulin therapy

8

- Oral medication
- Combination therapy
- Insulin therapy

Oral medication

Healthy eating through modification of food intake may be sufficient to achieve the aims of treatment in type 2 diabetes.

If symptoms persist and blood glucose levels remain elevated, oral medication may be required in addition to the dietary recommendations suggested.

Information regarding oral medication should include the following:

- The name of the drug
- The dose to be taken
- When to take the drug (i.e. before or at meal times)
- Hypoglycaemic effect of the drug (sulphonylureas)
- Side effects of the drug
- Possible interactions with other drugs taken
- What to do if problems occur (i.e. contact doctor or practice nurse)
- How to obtain prescription exemption (form FP92A, to be signed by a doctor).

Oral hypoglycaemic agents

There are five groups of drugs used in the treatment of type 2 diabetes:

- sulphonylureas
- biguanides
- postprandial glucose regulators (PPGRs)
- thiazolidinediones.
- glucosidase inhibitors.

The thiazolinediones were introduced in 1997. These drugs increase insulin sensitivity and lower triglyceride levels.

Sulphonylureas

Action
■ They stimulate release of insulin from the pancreas.

Usage
■ Sulphonylureas should be used in principle for people with type 2 diabetes of normal weight who are unable to achieve control of blood glucose levels by diet modification.

■ Sulphonylureas are potent drugs – and can cause profound hypoglycaemia which may be fatal. This problem is most common with the use of glibenclamide (particularly where it is used in elderly people or those with renal dysfunction).

■ Should hypoglycaemia occur, the drug should be substantially reduced or withdrawn.

■ Glibenclamide is a widely used sulphonylurea. It can, however, cause *significant hypoglycaemia*, particularly in elderly people or those with renal dysfunction.

Table 8.1 Sulphonylureas

Drug	Tablet strength (mg)	Dose (mg)
Glibenclamide (Daonil, Euglucon)	2.5 or 5	2.5–15 (once daily or divided doses)
Gliclazide (Diamicron, Minodiab)	80	40–320 daily (80 mg daily as single daily dose; higher doses as required)
Glimepiride (Amaryl)	1, 2, 3 or 4	1–6 (once daily after or with first meal of the day)
Glipizide (Glibenese)*	5	2.5–40 daily (15 mg as single daily dose; higher doses as required)
Gliquidone (Glurenorm)*	30	15–18 daily (up to 60 mg as single dose with breakfast; higher dose divided with meals)
Tolazamide (Tolanase)*	100 or 250	100–1,000 daily
Tolbutamide (Rastinon)*	500	500–2,000 daily (divided doses)

Note: as insulin is anabolic, the use of sulphonylureas (Table 8.1) may be associated with weight gain.

* These drugs are used rarely.

- Glimepiride is a long-lasting sulphonylurea. Its advantage is that all tablets are single dose.
- Gliclazide is perhaps the most commonly used. It is excreted in the bile and can therefore be used in renal insufficiency. It is less prone to cause hypoglycaemia in elderly people.
- Tolbutamide is safe and effective (particularly in elderly people) – although the tablets are large and may be difficult to swallow.

Cautions and contraindications
- Sulphonylureas can encourage weight gain
- Should not be used in pregnancy
- Should not be used during breast-feeding
- Should be used with caution in elderly people (because of dangers of hypoglycaemia)
- Should be used with caution – see above – in those with renal impairment.

Note: gliquidone and gliclazide may be used in renal impairment because they are metabolised and inactivated in the liver.

Side effects
- Usually mild and infrequent
- Gastrointestinal disturbances
- Headache
- Sensitivity reactions (rashes)
- Blood disorders (rare), e.g. thrombocytopenia, agranulocytosis and aplastic anaemia.

Biguanides

Action
- Unclear, but appear to decrease formation of glucose (gluconeogenesis).
- Increases peripheral utilisation of glucose.

Note that (1) metformin very rarely causes hypoglycaemia (except in large overdoses) and (2) metformin does not encourage weight gain.

Usage
The use of biguanides in the UK is shown in Table 8.2.
- Metformin is the first line of treatment in the person with type 2 diabetes.
- Metformin should be taken with food to minimise side effects, which may affect 30% of those treated with the drug.
- Side effects are less troublesome if small doses are used initially.

Table 8.2 Use of biguanides in the UK

Drug	Tablet strength (mg)	Dose (mg)
Metformin (Glucophage)	500 or 850	500–3,000 daily (divided doses with or after meals)

■ Patients rarely feel better when treated with metformin. Their well-being sometimes improves after withdrawal of the drug.

■ Risks of lactic acidosis have been exaggerated. These risks are considerably reduced if metformin is avoided in the presence of hepatic, renal or cardiac disease.

Cautions and contraindications

■ Lactic acidosis (potentially fatal): however, this almost always only occurs where metformin is used in people with renal failure.

■ Metformin should not be used in:
   ◆ renal failure
   ◆ hepatic failure
   ◆ heart failure
   ◆ alcoholism
   ◆ pregnancy
   ◆ breast-feeding.

Side effects

■ Diarrhoea
■ Epigastric discomfort/pain
■ Nausea
■ Anorexia
■ Unpleasant metallic taste
■ Vomiting
■ Constipation
■ Lactic acidosis (immediate withdrawal of drug)
■ Decreased vitamin B_{12} absorption.

Postprandial glucose regulators (PPGRs)

Action

■ PPGRs (e.g. repaglinide) work like a sulphonylurea, i.e. stimulate release of insulin from the pancreas and increase sensitivity of peripheral tissue to circulating insulin.

Table 8.3 Postprandial glucose regulators (PPGRs)

Drug	Tablet strength (mg)	Dose (mg)
Repaglinide (NovoNorm)	0.5, 1 or 2	Up to 16 daily (take one dose with one meal; maximum single dosage of 4 mg)

■ PPGRs have a faster onset and shorter duration of action than sulphonylureas.

Usage
The usage of PPGRs in the UK (repaglinide) is shown in Table 8.3.
■ PPGRs (e.g. repaglinide) are taken immediately before a meal.
■ If a meal is missed then it is not necessary to take a dose.
■ It can be introduced when diet and exercise are no longer adequate.
■ It can be used when metformin monotherapy is insufficient.
■ Incidence of hypos is less with repaglinide than with sulphonylureas.

Cautions and contraindications
■ Any known hypersensitivity to repaglinide or any of its derivatives.
■ Repaglinide should not be used in:
  ◆ type 1 diabetes
  ◆ diabetic ketoacidosis
  ◆ pregnancy or breast-feeding
  ◆ children aged < 12 years
  ◆ severe renal or hepatic function disorders.

Side effects
■ Hypoglycaemia
■ Transient visual disturbances
■ Gastrointestinal disturbances
■ Isolated cases of increases in liver enzymes
■ Hypersensitivity reactions.

A new class of amino acid derivative
Nateglinide (Starlix) is the first of a new class of amino acid derivatives that mimics the body's natural response to mealtime glucose. Launched by Novartis in May 2001, this drug helps control blood glucose levels by restoring a more physiological pattern of mealtime insulin release. In type 2 diabetes, there is a fundamental defect in the ability to release insulin immediately after meals, as a result of β-cell failure, which results in mealtime glucose 'spikes'. These

mealtime glucose 'spikes' are a significant contributor to cardiovascular disease, the major cause of death in people with type 2 diabetes. The activity of the drug is determined by the ambient blood glucose level – it is glucoresponsive, so it minimises the risk of hypoglycaemia. Clinical trials demonstrate its particular effectiveness in lowering glycated haemoglobin when it is used in combination with metformin therapy.

Action
- Enables mealtime insulin release
- Reduces post-meal glucose excursions
- Reduces glycated haemoglobin (HbA1c)
- Hypoglycaemia risk minimal.

Usage
- Licensed for use as both monotherapy and in combination with metformin
- Should be taken 30 minutes before meals
- Starting dose 60 mg before meals
- Maintenance dose 120 mg before meals.

Side effects
- Minimal hypoglycaemia
- Minimal weight gain (only 0.17 kg over 6 months when used in combination with metformin).

Thiazolidinediones

Action
- The thiazolidinediones (glitazones) act by reducing insulin resistance.
- They are both a first-line and an add-on treatment.
- They reduce blood glucose and insulin levels by increasing the effectiveness of available insulin in the liver, fat and muscle.
- They potentiate the action of both the body's own insulin and also injected insulin.

Usage
The usage of thiazolidinediones in the UK is shown in Table 8.4.
- Thiazolidinediones (glitazones) are licensed by NICE to be used in combination with either metformin or the sulphonylureas (but not both). Not licensed for use with insulin yet.
- The glitazones are well tolerated and, because of their mechanism of action, cannot cause hypos when given alone (i.e. as a first-line treatment).

Table 8.4 Thiazolidinediones (glitazones)

Drug	Tablet strength (mg)	Dose (mg)
Rosiglitazone (Avandia)	4, 8	4–8 daily (taken as single dose at any time)
Pioglitazone (Actos)	15, 30	15 or 30 once daily (in combination with metformin or a sulphonylurea, with or without food)

■ Pioglitazone is used only in combination with either metformin in obese patients or a sulphonylurea in patients with intolerance of or contraindications for metformin.

Cautions and contraindications
■ Rosiglitazone should not be used in:
  ◆ pregnancy or breast-feeding
  ◆ hepatic impairment or severe renal insufficiency.
■ Pioglitazone should not be used in:
  ◆ monotherapy
  ◆ children and adolescents
  ◆ pregnancy or breast-feeding
  ◆ patients with hypersensitivity to the drug, or those with heart failure or a history of heart failure or liver impairment.

Side effects
In combination with metformin:
■ Common side effects are:
  ◆ anaemia
  ◆ weight increase
  ◆ headache
  ◆ arthralgia
  ◆ haematuria
  ◆ impotence.
■ Uncommon side effects are:
  ◆ flatulence.
In combination with a sulphonylurea:
■ Common side effects are:
  ◆ weight increase
  ◆ dizziness
  ◆ flatulence.

Table 8.5 Oral hypoglycaemic drugs – interactions with other drugs

Drugs affected	Drug interacting	Effect
Oral hypoglycaemic drugs	Alcohol, β blockers, monoamine oxidase inhibitors, clofibrate, bezafibrate, gemfibrozil, fenofibrate	Hypoglycaemic effect increased
	Corticosteroids, bumetanide, furosemide (frusemide), thiazides and oral contraceptives	Hyperglycaemic effect increased (antagonistic)
	Lithium	May impair glucose tolerance
Sulphonylureas (tolbutamide)	Chloramphenicol, co-trimoxazole miconazole, fluconazole	Hypoglycaemic effect increased
Gliquidone, tolbutamide	Rifampicin	Reduced effect
Metformin	Alcohol	Increased risk of lactic acidosis
	Cimetidine	Increased plasma concentration of metformin
PPGRs (repaglinide)	β Blockers, monoamine oxidase inhibitors, ACE inhibitors, NSAIDs, salicylates, anabolic steroids, oral contraceptives, thiazides, corticosteroids, thyroid hormones, sympathomimetics	Interactions are not significant
Thiazolidinediones (rosiglitazone, pioglitazone)	Insulin – not licensed for use in the UK anyway	

- Uncommon side effects are:
  - glycosuria, hypoglycaemia, increase in LDH, appetite increase
  - headache, vertigo
  - abnormal vision
  - sweating
  - proteinuria
  - fatigue.

α-Glucosidase inhibitors

α-Glucosidase inhibitors (acarbose) block α-glucosidase enzymes, inhibiting carbohydrate digestion, thereby delaying the digestive process, so that glucose is absorbed through the colon.

The side effects of abdominal distension, malodorous flatulence and diarrhoea occur only when doses are started too high and increased too quickly. Unpleasant side effects may also occur if the patient is indulging in a glucose-rich diet.

Usage
Tablet strength is 50 mg or 100 mg; dose is 50 mg or 100 mg three times daily with meals.

Cautions and contraindications
- Gastrointestinal disease.

Unwanted effects
- Flatulence
- Abdominal distension
- Diarrhoea.

To minimise risks of unwanted effects, acarbose should be prescribed in low doses slowly increased over several weeks until optimal blood glucose levels are achieved (as discussed and agreed with the person concerned). It can be taken on a start low, go slow regimen: in weeks 1/2, 50 mg is taken with the first mouthful of food once daily; in weeks 3/4, 50 mg is taken twice daily; and in weeks 5/6, 50 mg is taken three times daily. After this the dosage is increased or titrated up to 100 mg three times daily dependent on the clinical response; this is the normal maintenance dose. During this period patients should also adhere to their dietary guidelines.

Combination therapy

Combination therapy can mean combinations of different oral hypoglycaemic agents (i.e. different tablets) or combinations of tablets and insulin. The combination of thiazolidinediones and a sulphonylurea or metformin has been dealt with in the section above because pioglitazone can be given only in combination (i.e. not as a monotherapy).

- As type 2 diabetes is a progressive disease, people with diabetes need increasing doses of tablets, extra drugs and eventually insulin to maintain good glucose control.
- Any combination of sulphonylurea, metformin and/or a glitazone is acceptable.
- The usual combination is a sulphonylurea with metformin or a glitazone.
- Metformin causes gastrointestinal side effects and people often feel better after starting insulin.
- People with diabetes often have other risk factors, such as hypertension or raised lipids, and need to take additional tablets to reduce these risks.
- The UKPDS demonstrated the importance of tight blood glucose control. Thus patients with HbA1c > 7.5% on a combination of tablets should consider the need for insulin.
- Tablet boxes to organise daily medication are available from chemists.

Combination therapy: sulphonylureas and metformin

- Combination therapy (of sulphonylureas and metformin) could be used where the person with type 2 diabetes has been unable to achieve control of blood glucose levels on maximum doses of sulphonylureas or metformin.
- This decision may be difficult and, in the interests of the person concerned, referral to a hospital diabetologist may be appropriate.
- The overweight person may 'improve control' when sulphonylureas are added to existing metformin therapy – at the expense of further weight increase.
- The person of normal weight who is hyperglycaemic on the maximum dose of a sulphonylurea may have metformin added to no good purpose, thereby delaying the use of insulin therapy which is urgently needed.

Combination therapy: insulin and tablets

- Traditionally, people with type 2 diabetes have been treated with tablets for as long as possible and then changed over to insulin.
- A new and acceptable approach is combination therapy with tablets and insulin.

- This helps people become accustomed to insulin injections and to adjusting the dose according to their blood glucose tests.
- Start by adding a long-acting insulin at bedtime (say 10 units) and monitoring the early morning glucose.
- The final dose of insulin needed to achieve a morning glucose < 6 mmol/l will depend mainly on body weight.
- The dose of insulin should be increased steadily until the target is achieved.
- Sulphonylureas or metformin should be continued at the previous dose, which should be more effective if the fasting glucose is well controlled.
- Glitazones are effective in combination with insulin, but are not licensed for such use in the UK.
- As the β cells in the pancreas cease to function, daytime blood glucose levels will creep up with a rise in HbA1c.
- At some stage, tablets have little useful effect and the person will have to move over to two or more daily injections of insulin.

Note that, at each stage in this process, the person with diabetes and the clinic team must decide whether or not to move on to the next stage. Many people, particularly if elderly or very overweight, may be better off accepting less than ideal metabolic control. In the UKPDS, the benefits of tight control were not seen for about 6 years. So, in people with a life expectancy shorter than this, there is no point in struggling for perfection.

Insulin therapy

Approximately 40% of people with type 2 diabetes subsequently require treatment with insulin for the following reasons:

- Insulin is obviously needed (where symptoms persist and blood glucose levels are high)
- Continuing weight loss (which may be gradual)
- Persistent ketonuria
- Blood glucose levels are high: HbA1c > 7.5%
- In the presence of intercurrent illness.

Where insulin is obviously needed, where symptoms persist, blood glucose levels are high, weight loss has continued and ketonuria persists, the decision is clear. The introduction of insulin therapy will almost always relieve symptoms, lower blood glucose levels and improve well-being.

Where intercurrent illness occurs, insulin will be required for the following reasons (and others):

- Infections
- Increased insulin resistance
- Deteriorating blood glucose control
- Steroid therapy (increasing doses)
- Myocardial infarction.

Note: after recovery, insulin is usually withdrawn and normal treatment recommenced.

Trial of insulin

- A 3-month trial of insulin may improve well-being and blood glucose levels in some people:
  - ◆ whose weight is stable
  - ◆ who are unable to achieve targets for blood glucose control appropriate for their age or for other reasons.
- After a 3-month trial of insulin the person concerned should choose whether to return to oral medication or remain on insulin therapy.
- Where the person with diabetes is overweight and poor blood glucose control persists, a decision to commence insulin therapy is more difficult.
- Further modification of the diet is necessary.
- A trial of insulin may be indicated, although in poorly controlled, overweight people, whose food intake is excessive, gross obesity may result.

Aims for therapy

In younger people with type 2 diabetes

The aim of treatment should be to improve blood glucose levels to reduce the risks of long-term complications.

In older people with type 2 diabetes (especially elderly people)

The aim of treatment should be to improve health and well-being.

Starting insulin therapy for people with type 2 diabetes

- The person concerned will require considerable support, education and careful management.
- Specialist help (the hospital team) may be required, if the primary care team are inexperienced in starting insulin therapy.
- An individual programme is required for stabilisation and continuing education.

- Blood sugar monitoring is almost always required if insulin therapy is commenced, replacing urine testing – if previously used (see Chapter 9).
- Assessment of the capability, lifestyle and wishes of the patient is important when starting insulin, so that the insulin regimen allows a desired and appropriate lifestyle.
- A long-acting insulin once daily, intermediate-acting insulin twice daily or pre-mixed insulin twice daily may be used for older people.
- Visual aids and 'automatic' injectors may be required – if so, the hospital team should be consulted.
- Insulin pens/needles are available on prescription.

Insulin sources

- Insulin is extracted from pork and beef pancreases and purified by crystallisation.
- Insulin can also be made biosynthetically by recombinant DNA technology using *Escherichia coli*.
- Insulin can also be produced semi-synthetically by modification of pork insulin.
- Human insulin (**emp**): insulin produced by enzyme modification of porcine insulin, sometimes known as semi-synthetic human insulin.
- Human insulin (**prb**): proinsulin recombinant bacteria, produced from proinsulin by genetic modification.
- Human insulin (**pyr**): insulin produced from a precursor obtained from a yeast genetically modified by recombinant DNA technology.

About insulin

- Insulin plays a key role in the body's regulation of carbohydrate, fat and protein metabolism.
- Diabetes mellitus is caused by a deficiency in insulin synthesis and secretion.
- Insulin is inactivated by gastrointestinal enzymes and must therefore be given by injection.
- It is usually injected into the upper arms, thighs, buttocks or abdomen (there may be increased absorption from a limb site after strenuous exercise).
- Insulin is usually administered subcutaneously using a syringe and needle.
- Portable injection devices (e.g. NovoPen, BD Pen Ultra, Penject) hold insulin in cartridge form. The dose can be 'clicked up' and shown on a dial. Disposable pen injection devices such as the Human Mixtard 30 Pen hold a larger reservoir of insulin and can be thrown away when empty. Each pen usually lasts a week, but this depends on the dosage used.

8

- Pen devices allow greater flexibility of lifestyle although more injections are required where a multiple dose regimen is used.
- A new insulin delivery device that is not a pen has been launched by Novo Nordisk (Innovo).
- Insulin can be given by continuous subcutaneous infusion (an insulin pump).
- When treating diabetic ketoacidosis, insulin should be given by intramuscular or intravenous injection, as absorption from subcutaneous sites can be slow and erratic.
- Minor allergic reactions at injection sites during the first few weeks of treatment are uncommon, usually transient and require no treatment.
- Rotation of injection sites lessens the chances of lipohypertrophy/lipoatrophy.
- Certain sites may become 'favoured' as their continued use lessens the discomfort of the injection.
- Insulin doses are determined on an individual basis (about 0.5–0.8 unit/kg body weight).
- Initial doses are small and gradually increased to avoid hypoglycaemia.

There are five main types of insulin preparation:

1. Those of short duration which have a relatively rapid onset of action, namely soluble forms of insulin, e.g. Human Actrapid, Humulin S, Human Velosulin. These can be given intramuscularly (i.m.) or intravenously (i.v.).
2. Those with an intermediate action, e.g. isophane insulin, insulin zinc suspension sometimes used for longer periods.
3. Mixtures of short and intermediate (isophane) insulins. These give a biphasic response, e.g. Human Mixtard 30/70. This is the largest group.
4. Those whose action is slower in onset and lasts for long periods, e.g. Human Ultratard.
5. Insulin analogues (see below).

Note: the duration of action of different insulin preparations varies considerably from one person to another and should be individually assessed before any dose adjustments are made. The monthly *MIMS Index* (Haymarket Press) contains a chart giving the onset, peak activity and duration of action of insulins.

Management of the side effects of insulin (prevention of hypoglycaemia)

- Hypoglycaemia may not be regarded as a side effect of insulin, because its hypoglycaemic action is therapeutic and normoglycaemia is the goal of treatment.

- Although hypoglycaemia may be defined as a blood glucose level < 4 mmol/l, symptoms of hypoglycaemia may be experienced when blood glucose levels are higher than this. Symptoms of hunger, light-headedness and tingling may be experienced as blood glucose levels are falling (from previously high levels), e.g. from 28 mmol/l to 11 mmol/l. Prevention of hypoglycaemia in efforts to achieve normoglycaemia includes the following in clinical management.

Insulin species

- Changing species of insulin may cause problems. Where people have been treated with animal (porcine and bovine) insulin for many years, and then changed over to 'human' insulin, the daily dose requires reduction by 10% or more. Human insulin appears to have profound hypoglycaemic action when used by such people. Although this has not yet been proven scientifically, subjective changes should not be taken lightly. Likewise, it is reported by people with diabetes that the warning signs of hypoglycaemia are also 'reduced' when their species of insulin is changed from 'animal' or 'natural' (porcine and bovine) to 'human'.
- Should hypoglycaemia or loss of warnings of hypoglycaemia occur, the patient's insulin should be changed back from human to the animal species with due understanding. Close blood glucose monitoring is essential where any change of insulin is made.
- A choice of insulin species is now available for people with diabetes. This choice is also included in the insulin delivery systems that accompany the insulins in use, i.e. pens, syringes, needles, vials and cartridges of insulin. Note that syringes, insulin vials and cartridges, pen needles and pens are available on FP10 prescription forms.
- It is important that the *species* of insulin is recorded and that any change of insulin *species* is recorded. The person with diabetes should know his or her own insulin *species*.

Insulin type

- This refers to the hypoglycaemic action of a particular insulin and may be associated with its name.
- The hypoglycaemic action of insulin refers to: *onset* of action; *rise* of action; *peak* of action; *fall* of action; and *duration* of action (Fig. 8.1).
- The onset, rise, peak, fall and duration of insulin effect are considered when insulin is prescribed. The prescription will relate to the person's glycaemic state, lifestyle (eating habits, activity levels) and medical state. Close blood glucose monitoring is required where any change in insulin type is made.
- It is important that the *type* of insulin is recorded and that any change of insulin *type* is recorded. The person with diabetes should also know his or her own insulin *type*.

8

Fig. 8.1 Hypoglycaemic action of insulin

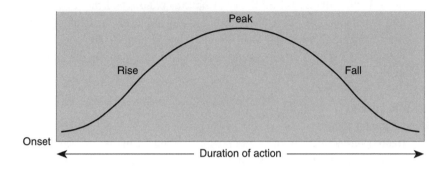

Insulin analogues: short-acting insulin analogues, e.g. lispro, have a short duration effect and can be injected at or just before meal times. This effect deals with the postprandial glucose peak. Lasts about 2 hours

Insulin dose

■ This will vary after stabilisation and will relate to the glycaemic state, lifestyle (eating habits and activity levels), medical state and the insulin regimen desired by the person with diabetes. In addition glycated haemoglobin levels and day-to-day glucose levels are discussed with the person concerned. In this way, the person with diabetes is engaged in all discussions and decisions relating to his or her own diabetes control and care.

■ It is important that the *dose* of insulin is recorded and that any change in insulin *dose* is recorded. The person with diabetes should also know his or her own insulin *dose*.

Note: for further information regarding the detection, prevention and treatment of hypoglycaemia, see Chapter 9 (page 125).

Guideline for teaching self-administration of insulin

Ideally, the person with diabetes requiring insulin therapy should have access to the hospital team. Considerable time, support, education and out of hours telephone contact/home visiting will be required initially and in a staged continuing process until confidence is gained and blood glucose levels stabilised.

Training and experience in 'starting' people on insulin therapy are required. Should there be no specialist team available and insulin therapy is indicated in an older person with diabetes the following guideline is provided; further points on education required are provided in Chapters 13 and 14.

The following steps are required:

- Assessment of the person with diabetes
- Preparation and support
- Understanding the equipment
- Drawing up insulin
- Giving the injection
- Care of equipment
- Prevention of hypoglycaemia
- Treatment of hypoglycaemia
- Contact telephone number
- Identification
- Anticipation of problems and questions
- Evaluating learning.

Assessment

Language	For communication
Literacy	Understanding written material

Culture ⎤
Home, work, social conditions ⎦ Lifestyle

Hearing ⎤
Sight |
Other medical problems |
Physical state ⎬ Physical ability
Mobility |
Dexterity ⎦

Mental state ⎤
Intellect |
Preconceived ideas ⎬ Mental and emotional state
Fear factor ⎦

Preparation and support required

It is important to take into account preconceived ideas and fear (particularly of the needle). Emphasise the benefits of insulin, improved well-being and that support is available.

The benefits of insulin

■ Direct action
■ No need to take tablets (for diabetes)
■ Feel better
■ Improved lifestyle
■ Lower blood glucose levels
■ Risks of complications reduced.

A 'dummy' injection

Experience of a 'dummy' injection by the nurse/doctor as well as the person with diabetes can be useful. Many people imagine the needle to be large and that it is inserted into a vein. It may be helpful for the person concerned to meet another patient who has successfully transferred to insulin treatment.

An optimistic, helpful and positive approach is essential.

Understanding the equipment

The equipment includes insulin (bottle or cartridges), syringes (pen devices/ needles), cotton wool, needle clipper (discuss container for syringe disposal), and educational material (leaflets on drawing up and giving insulin).

Insulin bottle or cartridges

Teach
■ Name, species and type
■ Action – peak – duration
■ Dose
■ Expiry date
■ Storage (bottle in use – spare bottle in fridge); pen devices should not be kept in fridge)
■ Spare bottles/cartridges in fridge
■ Prescription (check exemption).

Syringes (pen devices/needles)

Teach
■ Take to pieces
■ Show how they work

- Explain types of syringe/markings (50 units – 0.5 ml/100 units – 1 ml)
- Demonstrate pen device/needle – correctly fitting together
- Air bubbles – how to expel
- Storage and re-use (one syringe/pen needle may be used for several doses)
- Prescription (required).

Cotton wool

Teach
- Supplied by the person with diabetes
- Tissues may be used
- Used for gentle massage after injection.

Needle clipper

Teach
- Demonstrate
- Disposal
- Replacement (obtained from GP or hospital clinic)
- Prescription (required).

Disposal of sharps
This depends on whether the local authority and/or local hospital clinic/GP has arrangements for collecting sharps boxes. Most areas do not have this facility, in which case diabetes patients should use their B-D Safe-Clip device to snap off the needle from the syringe, putting it into an opaque plastic container that is then screwed tightly shut; this is then sealed with strong tape for additional safety and disposed of with the household waste. Lancets should be disposed of in the same way, ensuring that the point of the lancet is pressed firmly into the cover first. Used insulin bottles and cartridges should be wrapped up and disposed of in domestic waste.

Educational material

- Written leaflets
- Pictorial information.

Drawing up insulin

Teach
- The correct dose (write this down)
- How to draw up insulin correctly
- How to expel air bubbles

- When to give injection (20–30 min pre-meal, except for lispro, which is given immediately after food)
- Written leaflets (see resources list, Appendix VIII).

Giving the injection

Teach
- The angle of injection should relate to the length of the needle used, e.g. the shorter the needle length, the more acute the angle
- Check dexterity (right or left handed; use of hands)
- Sites/rotation (insulin absorbed more quickly from abdominal site or in limbs following exercise) (Fig. 8.2)
- Site for injection relaxed
- Massage gently with cotton wool/syringe after injection
- Encourage quick needle insertion (less uncomfortable)
- Encourage steady depression of plunger when injecting insulin
- Written and illustrated leaflets (see resources list, Appendix VIII)
- Discuss the effects of too many injections in one small area of injection site, e.g. poor absorption, reduced insulin effectiveness – lipohypertrophy (human insulin), lipoatrophy (animal insulin).

Fig. 8.2 Site rotation chart

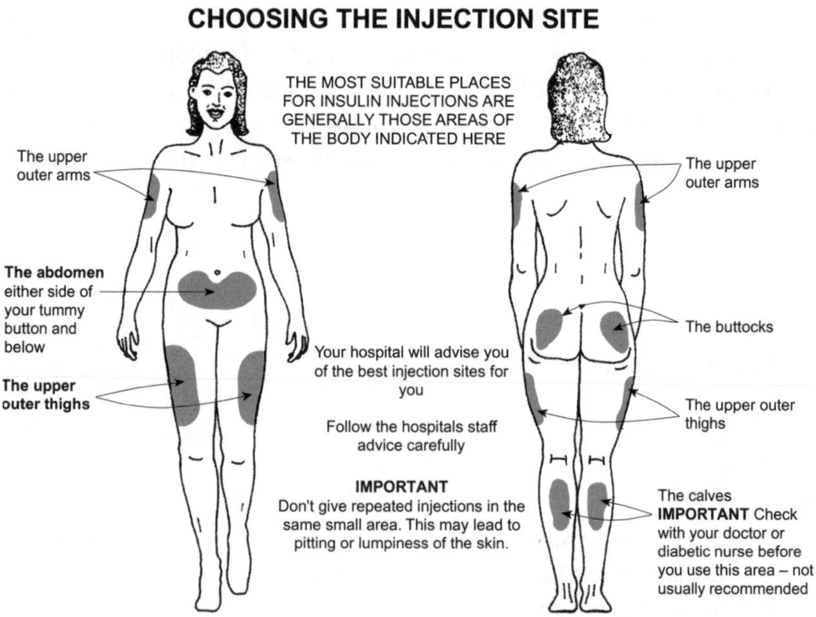

CHOOSING THE INJECTION SITE

THE MOST SUITABLE PLACES FOR INSULIN INJECTIONS ARE GENERALLY THOSE AREAS OF THE BODY INDICATED HERE

The upper outer arms

The abdomen either side of your tummy button and below

The upper outer thighs

Your hospital will advise you of the best injection sites for you

Follow the hospitals staff advice carefully

IMPORTANT
Don't give repeated injections in the same small area. This may lead to pitting or lumpiness of the skin.

The upper outer arms

The buttocks

The upper outer thighs

The calves
IMPORTANT Check with your doctor or diabetic nurse before you use this area – not usually recommended

Care of equipment

Teach
- Keep all together (with other equipment, e.g. for monitoring)
- Always have a spare insulin (keep in fridge) bottle or cartridges
- Keep away from children
- List equipment required before attending surgery or hospital clinic – check insulin species, name, types of syringes used
- Re-use of syringes (pen device needles)
- Correct disposal (syringe/pen device needles, insulin vials and cartridges).

Prevention of hypoglycaemia

Teach
- Note that exercise, alcohol and sexual activity may lower blood glucose levels sufficiently to cause hypoglycaemia
- Eat regularly (meals and snacks)
- Do not delay or miss meals
- Check dietary advice (refer to dietitian)
- Take correct dose of insulin
- Eat more carbohydrate (if activity increased)
- Less insulin needed (if strenuous activity anticipated)
- Note: monitoring and education are required for self-adjustment of insulin
- Carry glucose tablets/sweets – always (keep in car – if driving)
- Inform DVLA – if a driver (new to insulin)
- Carry identification (necklace, bracelet or card) (see resources list, Appendix VIII).

Treatment of hypoglycaemia

Teach
- Recognition of symptoms (pallor, sweating, etc.)
- Take 2–3 glucose tablets/sweet drink/sweets
- Follow-up with substantial snack/meal high in carbohydrate
- Do not count this snack/meal in (it is extra to usual meals)
- Use of glucagon (by relative/friend – if unconscious)
- If driving – slow down, stop car safely – remove keys from ignition – move to passenger seat – treat as above
- Note possible reasons for hypoglycaemia:
  ? too much insulin
  ? insufficient food
  ? delayed meal
  ? more activity

? stress
? hot weather
? new injection site used.

Note: if hypoglycaemic episodes occur frequently and/or regularly, extra blood tests should be carried out to establish whether any pattern causes them (e.g. extra activity or too much insulin).
Note: there may (often) be no reason.

Contact telephone number

Teach
■ Surgery number
■ Hospital diabetes centre/clinic number
■ Out of hours number.

Identification

Teach
■ Importance of personal ID
■ Availability and source for necklace/bracelet (local jewellers or see resources list, Appendix VIII)
■ Identification cards (Diabetes UK/insulin companies – see resources list, Appendix VIII).

Anticipation of problems and questions

Examples

Human insulin – does it come from humans?
■ Reassure that this is not so. This may reflect concerns about AIDS (see section 'About insulin' earlier in this chapter).

'Forgetting' the injection: what should I do?
■ Advise – wait to give the next one, or two doses may be given close together (a hypoglycaemic reaction could result).

Giving the wrong dose (too much or too little)?
■ Explain action/peak/duration of insulin
■ Explain effects of too much insulin – hypoglycaemia – recognition and treatment

- Explain effects of too little insulin – hyperglycaemia – correct at next dose, or seek medical advice if blood glucose levels high (a quick acting dose may be required).

Spirit for cleaning the skin?
- This is not required
- Makes injections uncomfortable
- Toughens injection sites.

Bleeding after injection?
- Reassure this is nothing to worry about
- Check injection technique
- Apply gentle pressure to site if bleeding occurs.

Evaluating learning

- At each stage after demonstration and teaching the person with diabetes/relative should demonstrate understanding
- Practical skills should be demonstrated
- Understanding evaluated by appropriate questions and in discussion
- Follow-up appointments/home visits should be made at regular intervals until confidence is gained
- Monitoring is important once insulin therapy is commenced, in order to adjust insulin slowly to the appropriate level required for blood glucose levels, symptom relief and improved well-being
- Monitoring techniques require education and evaluation after the start of insulin therapy.

Further reading

Airey M, Williams R (2000). Hypoglycaemia induced by exogenous insulin 'human' and animal insulin compared. *Diabetic Medicine* July.

DCCT Research Group (1993). The effect of intensive treatment of diabetes on the development of long term complications in insulin-dependent diabetes mellitus. *N Engl J Med* **329**: 977–86.

The DECODE Study Group (1999). Glucose tolerance and mortality: comparison of WHO and American Diabetes Association diagnostic criteria. *Lancet* **354**: 617–21.

News and Information (2001). New treatment could cut cardiovascular risk for millions of diabetics worldwide. *Diabetes Today* 4(4): 111.

Kerr D, Everett J (1998). Role in the management of type 1 and type 2 diabetes. *Prescriber* 19 June: 45–9.

Patriell A (1998). Insulin therapy in type 1 and type 2 diabetes. *Prescriber* 19 June: 39–45.

The Research Unit, Royal College of Physicians, British Diabetic Association and Royal College of General Practitioners (1993). *Guidelines of good practice in the diagnosis and treatment of non-insulin-dependent diabetes mellitus.* London: RCP.

Timmins IG (1992). *Notes on Oral Hypoglycaemia Agents. Insulin Therapy.* Sheffield Health Authority.

UKPDS Study Group (1998). Intensive blood-glucose control with sulphonylureas or insulin compared with conventional treatment and risk of complications in patients with type 2 diabetes (UKPDS 33). *Lancet* **352**: 837–53.

Control of blood glucose levels

- Monitoring diabetes control by the primary care team
- High blood glucose levels (hyperglycaemia)
- Low blood glucose levels (hypoglycaemia)
- Self-monitoring in diabetes care

Monitoring diabetes control by the primary care team

- The monitoring of the person with diabetes by the primary care team should support and check self-monitoring as well as ascertaining the effectiveness of treatment.
- Targets for control should be negotiated and realistic.
- Long-term control can be confirmed by annual glycated haemoglobin or serum fructosamine tests.

Glycated haemoglobin (HbA1c)

The measurement of glycated haemoglobin is widely accepted as an objective and quantitative index of blood glucose levels during the preceding 6–10 weeks. This test is usually performed annually as an indicator of control over the period preceding the test. A fasting blood glucose level usually provides a similar result to the HbA1c test. HbA1c may be required more frequently where blood glucose control is poor. It should be remembered that the glycated haemoglobin test does not represent individual peaks and troughs in blood glucose levels. A low glycated haemoglobin or result within the normal range (4–8% depending on the laboratory range) may indicate good control, although not reflecting levels of hypoglycaemia. Individual self-test results are also important and should always be discussed in any review of blood glucose control.

Serum fructosamine

This is an objective and quantitative test reflecting blood glucose control over the preceding 2–3 weeks only. This test is thus less useful because its timespan is shorter. Fructosamine levels are used in some districts.

The benefits of monitoring

On diagnosis, after the start or change of therapy and at any review, checks should be made on symptoms experienced (if any), ketonuria, glycosuria and blood glucose levels.

Confirmation of improvement in blood glucose levels, especially in the absence of symptoms (in type 2 diabetes), will encourage continuity of self-care, treatment and monitoring.

Successful weight reduction will almost always improve blood glucose levels in type 2 diabetes.

The success/failure of oral medication can be confirmed and medication adjusted if necessary.

A decision regarding the initiation of insulin therapy can be made.

Monitoring of dietary habits, changes in weight, lifestyle and other medical problems is also essential (particularly in elderly people) as any or all of these may affect diabetes control, necessitating possible review and changes in treatment.

Monitoring by the practice team also involves urine testing for proteinuria, measurement of blood pressure, and examination and surveillance for complications of diabetes, e.g. visual deterioration, retinopathy, foot problems (see guidelines for follow-up and review in Chapter 6).

High blood glucose levels (hyperglycaemia)

Hyperglycaemia is generally regarded to exist where blood glucose levels are above 10 mmol/l. This is certainly correct in a younger person with diabetes. For women who are pregnant, blood glucose levels should not rise above 7 mmol/l even after meals.

In older people, however, especially where weight is a problem, blood glucose levels may be higher than 10 mmol/l. It is important that levels are discussed and that the person is symptom-free.

Hyperglycaemia may be caused by:

- Untreated diabetes
- Too much food   } these may occur on special occasions
- The wrong type of food
- Insufficient medication (incorrect dose)
- Insufficient insulin (incorrect dose)

- Overuse of particular injection sites
- Poor injection technique
- Reduction of activity
- Decreased mobility
- Infections/illness
- An increase in concurrent medication affecting glycaemic control (e.g. steroid therapy)
- Stress – life changes (retirement, bereavement)
- A weight increase.

Symptoms of hyperglycaemia need to be explained, such as thirst, polyuria, nocturia (incontinence in elderly people), lethargy, irritability and visual changes.

Suggested changes and action to be taken: if the person with diabetes is self-monitoring, it should be explained that occasional 'high' tests need not be acted upon. However, should hyperglycaemia persist, adjustments may be required (according to identified causes of the high blood sugar levels) regarding food/activity/medication/insulin. Particular action should be taken if an infection or illness disturbs blood glucose control.

Guidelines for management of illness (by the primary care team)

- Monitoring equipment such as Ketur Test and blood glucose test strips, e.g. Glucotrend (in date and kept in airtight containers in a dry place, not in a fridge) should be available in the surgery and in doctor's bag.
- Short-acting insulin (e.g. Human Actrapid) may be useful to lower blood glucose levels in acute illness (in surgery and in doctor's bag).

Guide for the physician

- Review therapy, check blood glucose levels and presence/absence of ketonuria, and treat intercurrent illness.
- Consider short-term insulin therapy (for people usually treated with diet and oral hypoglycaemic agents).
- Ketonuria unlikely in type 2 diabetes.
- Refer to hospital if vomiting/hyperglycaemia/ketosis persists.
- Blood glucose control may deteriorate rapidly during an illness of any kind. People with diabetes require instructions on action to be taken during any intercurrent illness (Table 9.1).
- It is helpful if the relative or carer is also aware of these instructions in case the person with diabetes is unable to carry them out.

- The relative or carer should be able to draw up and give insulin if necessary and be able to monitor blood or urine glucose levels (if this is possible and appropriate).
- The person with diabetes/relative should have an emergency contact telephone number.

Table 9.1 Illness rules: a guideline for the person with type 2 diabetes

- A minor illness, such as a cold, may cause your blood sugar levels to rise
- Blood sugar levels will return to normal once the infection is over, so usual treatment can then be resumed
- Consult your doctor if the illness persists, if you have symptoms of high sugar levels or if you have high tests
- Headaches and sore throats can safely be relieved using paracetamol or aspirin
- Sugar-free cough remedies are available from your local pharmacist
- Vomiting may result in you being unable to keep tablets down – consult your doctor
- Vomiting and diarrhoea may result in you losing a lot of fluid – consult your doctor
- You may need this fluid replaced
- You may need insulin for a short time

CONSULT YOUR DOCTOR

IMPORTANT RULES

- Continue with your diabetes treatment (diet and tablets or insulin)
- Ensure that you drink plenty of liquid (water, tea, etc.)
- Test urine or blood 24 hourly to check on how you are doing
- If you are not hungry, substitute meals with a liquid or light diet (soup, ice cream, glucose drinks, milk – see Table 9.2 for emergency exchange list)

Consult your doctor in good time.

Table 9.2 Food/fluids to substitute for portions when you are off your food

If you are ill and do not feel like eating, replace your normal food portions ('exchanges') with fluids such as milk, fruit juice or Lucozade. The list on page 129 gives you an idea of suitable substitutes.

You should also aim to drink plenty of sugar-free liquids (at least 5 pints each day).

Table 9.2 contd

Fluids to provide 10 grams of carbohydrate (i.e. one exchange or portion)

	Quantity
Lucozade, or similar glucose drink	50 ml/2 fl. oz
Fruit juices (natural, unsweetened)	100 ml/4 fl. oz (one wine glass)
Coke or Pepsi (not diet)	100 ml/4 fl. oz (one wine glass)
Lemonade, or similar carbonated drink	200 ml/7 fl. oz (one cup)
Milk	200 ml/7 fl. oz (one cup)
Soup (thickened, creamed, e.g. chicken)	200 ml/7 fl. oz (one cup)
Soup (tomato, tinned)	100 ml/4 fl. oz (one wine glass)

Foods to provide 10 grams of carbohydrate (i.e. one exchange or portion)

Ice-cream (plain)	50 g/2 oz (one scoop or small brickette)
Natural yoghurt	150 g/5 oz (one pot)
Low-fat, fruit or flavoured yoghurt	75 g/2.5 oz (half a pot)
Porridge oats, made with water	100 g/4 oz
Jelly (ordinary)	15 g/0.5 oz (two cubes)
Jelly (ordinary made up with water)	75 g/3 oz (one-eighth of the whole jelly or two tablespoonfuls)
Ready to serve custard	75 g/3 oz (one-sixth of a 425 g can)

Other useful carbohydrate-containing foods

Complan, 1 x 57 g sachet + 200 ml milk (made up as directed)	Contains 45 g carbohydrate
Ovaltine, 24 g (3–4 heaped teaspoons) + 200 ml milk	Contains 24 g carbohydrate
Horlicks, 25 g (3–4 heaped teaspoons) + 200 ml milk	Contains 29 g carbohydrate

When people feel nauseous it helps to find out what they would prefer to eat. The composition of foods is usually described on the packet. You are aiming to replace the carbohydrate in the food they would normally eat during the day. For example, some people find that foods such as 'Rice Cakes' are useful if they feel nauseous.

Low blood glucose levels (hypoglycaemia)

■ Hypoglycaemia is generally regarded to exist where blood glucose levels are below 3 mmol/l.

■ It is important to remember that symptoms of hypoglycaemia may be experienced at levels higher than 3 mmol/l, in particular where blood glucose levels have been high for a period of time (e.g. after diagnosis).

■ People with diabetes who strictly control their blood glucose levels are more at risk of hypoglycaemia.

■ Hypoglycaemia can be delayed (many hours after extra activity).

Hypoglycaemia may be caused by:

■ Too little food (especially in elderly people)
■ Delayed or missed meals
■ Increased medication or insulin
■ Increased activity (exercise)
■ Increased mobility
■ A decrease in concurrent medication affecting glycaemic control
■ Stress – life changes
■ Hot weather (insulin treated – insulin absorbed more rapidly)
■ Change of injection site (where one site has been used repeatedly followed by use of a new site)
■ A decrease in weight (particularly in elderly people)
■ The presence of renal failure
■ Alcohol use.

Symptoms of hypoglycaemia need to be explained, such as sweating, pallor, headache, tingling of the lips, pounding heart, blurred vision, irritability, lack of concentration (confusion).

Diminished warning signs

Warning signs may not occur:

■ In the presence of autonomic neuropathy, where diabetes has been diagnosed for many years (over 10 years).
■ Where strict blood glucose control exists.
■ Where repeated attacks of hypoglycaemia reduce significant symptoms.

The treatment of hypoglycaemia

Action to be taken

If the patient is conscious
■ Give a sugary drink (use a straw) or glucose sweets (3–4) or sweets
■ Give a substantial snack or meal (extra to normal meals) high in carbohydrate
■ Check that blood glucose levels have returned to normal.

If the patient is uncooperative
■ Use Hypostop gel (available on prescription)
■ Insert gel (about one-third of a bottle) orally and massage gently around cheeks (the gel is absorbed into the buccal mucosa)
■ *Once cooperative* – give a sugary drink or glucose tablets (3–4)
■ Give a substantial snack or meal (extra to normal meals) high in carbohydrate
■ Check that blood glucose levels have returned to normal.

If the patient is unconscious
■ Give glucagon injection (available on prescription)
■ Place patient in recovery position and await return of consciousness (about 15–20 minutes)
■ *On recovery,* sit patient up
■ Give a sugary drink (use a straw) or glucose sweets (3–4) or sweets
■ Give a substantial snack or meal (extra to normal meals) high in carbohydrate
■ Check that blood glucose levels have returned to normal.

Note:
1. Should glucagon not render the patient conscious:

CALL THE DOCTOR

or

EMERGENCY SERVICES – DIAL 999

2. Glucagon can cause vomiting.
3. The patient may feel very cold on regaining consciousness.

Self-monitoring in diabetes care

- When appropriate, after diagnosis and if they are able, people with diabetes should become accustomed to monitoring their own health.
- In a broad sense, this includes general health and well-being, diabetes control, eyesight, weight, dental care, care of the feet and footwear.
- In order to promote health and reduce risks of complications, the monitoring of diabetes control (urine/blood glucose levels) requires particular attention and involves careful assessment and education by the care team.
- Self-monitoring allows the person with diabetes to check his or her own control, take responsibility for his or her own condition and maintain independence (as far as possible).
- Four stages are required in the process of initiating a self-monitoring programme.

Stage I: assessment

Physical

Vision, colour vision, coordination and manual dexterity should be checked. If there are problems with any of these a partner, carer or the primary care team will need to monitor control.

Educational

Capability of understanding and retention of knowledge. Literacy, for back-up written material, language and culture.

Attitudinal

The desire to self-monitor and take responsibility for own control.

Lifestyle

Fitting self-monitoring in with home, work and social life.

User ability

Ability to understand and take action on test results.

Stage II: teaching

Teaching involves the person with diabetes/relative/carer:

- learning the skill
- recording the information gained
- understanding the information gained
- acting on the information where appropriate.

In addition:

- After an assessment, teaching should be adapted according to the needs of the individual and his or her capabilities.
- Explanations should be clear and in language that is understood.
- It should be recognised that some people will require more in-depth information.
- Numbers and times of tests should be negotiated.

Stage III: evaluation

- Record teaching and information given.
- Allow time for discussion of self-monitoring and to answer questions about recorded results.
- Check testing technique by asking the person with diabetes/relative/carer to demonstrate a test when attending the surgery for review.
- Check understanding of tests, interpretation of results and any action taken.

Stage IV: reinforcement

- On subsequent visits, ensure that monitoring is discussed.
- At least annually, check testing technique, understanding of tests, interpretation of results and any action taken.
- Show interest in tests and results.
- Be encouraging and supportive at all times.
- Do not make judgements on people who fail to carry out tests, record them or bring their records for review.
- Re-negotiate and encourage **always.**

Who is monitoring?

- The person with diabetes
- The relative
- The carer.

Why monitor?

- To indicate that diabetes is controlled using urine or blood tests so that urine/blood glucose levels remain within limits appropriate to the person's age, duration of diabetes, lifestyle and wishes (with the knowledge of risks of short-term and long-term complications of diabetes).
- To indicate deterioration of diabetes control, so that an appropriate treatment review can take place.
- To indicate improvement of diabetes control after a weight, dietary, medication or insulin change or adjustment.
- To appreciate the reasons for self-monitoring, the person with diabetes needs to understand the factors affecting the rise and fall of urine/blood glucose levels, including the associated symptoms, possible reasons, changes to be made and actions to be taken.
- Targets for testing and control should be appropriate and individually negotiated.

Urine testing

- Other than in children (to avoid excessive finger pricks), urine testing is of little use in type 1 diabetes.
- Urine testing is most commonly used in people with type 2 diabetes (elderly people, or in certain types of employment, where blood testing may be impossible to carry out).
- Urine testing is inexpensive.
- The meaning of urine tests must be individually explained to each patient.
- A freshly passed urine specimen pre-breakfast, after early morning voiding, will indicate control during the day.
- Tests taken about 2 hours after a meal (2 hours post-evening meal) will indicate urinary glucose levels at their highest.
- If the renal threshold is individually explained, using a freshly voided specimen and a finger-prick blood test (at the same time – in surgery), people with diabetes will understand the meaning of their own urine tests and their relationship with blood glucose levels.
- A negative (or trace of glycosuria) urine test is the aim for older people, unless the renal threshold is found to be low.

- The renal threshold is usually equivalent to 10 mmol/l (blood glucose). This level rises with age.
- Often older people show negative urine tests but have blood glucose levels of 17 mmol/l or more (a high renal threshold).
- A negative urine test will not indicate hypoglycaemia, which may occur when older people are treated with sulphonylurea therapy.
- Should hypoglycaemia be suspected (from discussion of symptoms or reports of 'dizzy do's') blood sugar levels should be checked and medication or insulin reduced.
- Correctly taught and timed urine dipstick tests are simpler and safer than urine tests using tablets, which are caustic, messy and may be incorrectly used.
- A watch or clock with a second hand is required for home urine testing.
- Urine testing strips are available on prescription (free – except for people treated with diet alone, under the ages of 60 and 65 years of age – women and men respectively).
- The person with diabetes should be taught how to record tests and provided with a testing diary (available free – see resources list, Appendix VIII). These may also be obtained from the hospital clinic or centre.

Blood testing

- Blood testing is essential for people with type 1 diabetes, pre-pregnancy, during pregnancy or for those with gestational diabetes.
- Blood testing should usually be used by people with type 2 diabetes, treated with insulin.
- Blood testing may be used for people with type 2 diabetes, treated with diet or oral hypoglycaemic agents.
- Blood testing may be the monitoring method of choice for anyone with diabetes.
- Where people with diabetes are unable to self-monitor or use urine tests, blood testing is useful, even essential, to form a picture of day-to-day diabetes control. In these cases blood testing should be carried out by a carer or by a member of the primary care team. Such occasions might be:
  - where control is poor
  - where a treatment change is indicated
  - to monitor a treatment change
  - where hypoglycaemia is suspected.

Blood testing technique
- It is essential that hands are washed (by the person testing), preferably in warm water to encourage blood flow to the finger tips and to ensure that the test is uncontaminated.

Fig. 9.1 There are many devices for blood glucose monitoring for people with diabetes, using a meter and test strips. This photograph shows the Accu-Chek Advantage (Roche Diagnostics).

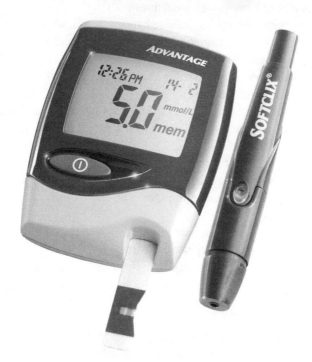

■ Spirit swabs should not be used to clean the skin as the spirit may affect results.
■ The side of the tips of fingers should be used (less painful).
■ Fingers used should be changed at each test (to avoid discomfort).
■ If the drop of blood is difficult to collect (into a 'tear' or 'tap' drop), Vaseline may be applied to the finger tip site before the test (this will accumulate the blood, stop it from spreading and will not affect the test).
■ Finger-pricking lancets can be re-capped and re-used.
■ Lancets, after use, should be re-capped and dropped into a capped container (they may then be disposed of in household waste, as indicated in Chapter 8, page 119, or according to local sharps disposal procedures).

Interpretation of results: action to take
■ Blood tests taken pre-meal and pre-bed will indicate control.
■ One blood test each day, taken at a different time, will provide a blood glucose profile over several days.
■ Pre-meal tests are the most useful, because post-meal tests will rise according to type of food eaten.

- A post-meal test can be useful in noting the effects of foods eaten.
- Blood tests should be carried out more frequently during the course of an infection or intercurrent illness (2–4 hourly).
- Should blood glucose levels be consistently high or low, reasons for this should be examined and appropriate action taken.
- Occasional high tests should not be acted upon unless they consistently occur at the same time of day.
- Should lifestyle be different on weekdays or weekends, blood tests will demonstrate this. Adjustments in food, medication or insulin may be required.
- If extra activity or exercise is anticipated, blood glucose levels should be checked beforehand and extra carbohydrate taken or insulin reduced (or both).
- After extra activity or exercise, blood glucose levels should be checked soon afterwards and some hours later (in case of delayed hypoglycaemia).
- Correctly taught and timed, visually read, blood testing strips are a sufficient guide to blood glucose levels.
- If the person with diabetes has poor vision or is colour blind, blood glucose meters (for use with their appropriate strips) are available for purchase (or loan from hospital clinics or centres), providing a numerical reading.
- Strip guides (for guiding blood onto the test patch) and talking meters are available for those who are blind.
- Meters should be suggested only in association with education about their use.
- Correct meter care and quality control are essential where meters are used for self-monitoring (as well as those used in a surgery).
- Blood monitoring strips are available on prescription (free – except for people treated with diet alone, under the ages of 60 and 65 years of age – women and men respectively).
- Finger-pricking devices may be obtained from hospital clinics or centres. Alternatively they can be purchased by the individual. They are not available on FP10.
- Finger-pricking lancets should be checked for their compatibility with the selected device.
- Recording of blood tests should be taught and a testing diary provided (available free – see resources list, Appendix VIII). These may also be obtained from the hospital clinic or centre.

Note: should there be any problems regarding self-monitoring using blood tests, interpretation of results, action to be taken or a blood glucose meter required, it is advisable to refer the person concerned to the local hospital clinic or diabetes centre.

References

Crawley H (1988). *Food Portion Sizes.* London: MAFF.
Davies J, Dickenson J (1991). *Nutrient Content of Food Portions.* London: RSC.

Eye care and screening

- A National Diabetes Retinal Screening Programme
- Features of an acceptable national programme: an integrated pattern of care
- Organisation of diabetic eye screening in primary care
- The role of the primary care team
- Visual acuity
- Opticians
- Fundoscopy

A National Diabetes Retinal Screening Programme

Guidance from the National Screening Committee/National Service Framework for Diabetes on retinal screening will be available by 2002, based on the recommendations of the Diabetes UK Advisory Panel to the UK National Screening Committee (2001) (website: www.diabetic-retinopathy.screening. nhs.uk/recommendations.html).

Summary of recommendations

- It is now a practical possibility to introduce a national risk reduction programme to preserve the sight of people with diabetes.
- A programme would need to be rolled out over a period of 3–4 years as funding and trained staff become available.
- It is estimated that about 1,000 optometrists across the UK are currently involved in diabetic retinopathy monitoring, but not all in systematic programmes.
- A regular (annual) eye surveillance programme of all people with diabetes will bring about a reduction of sight loss from diabetic retinopathy.
- A national scheme must eventually meet the following criteria:
  - ◆ annual programme for all those with diabetes
  - ◆ quality assurance written into the service

- ◆ the preferred method is digital imaging
- ◆ the programme integrated with the pattern of care for people with diabetes.
- There are a large number of surveillance initiatives, which currently provide services, not all of which meet the required specifications. It is important that the introduction of a national scheme does not disadvantage these existing schemes, but allows their enhancement to the approved higher specifications.
- Involving clients and providers in the local organisation of schemes will help to encourage a high take-up.
- The programme must be accessible to all those patients with diabetes, whether they are cared for in the community or in secondary care.
- Patients should not be expected to travel long distances to diabetes centres to be screened.
- The programme should be flexible enough to provide easy access for all patients and may encompass services provided in diabetes centres, in the community at primary care premises or other convenient locations, mobile vans and high street optometrists.

Screening methods

- Ophthalmoscopy and retinal photography with subsequent grading are the two main approaches used.
- Digital fundus photography has replaced slide and Polaroid photography.
- Digital photography facilitates the taking and storing of photographs and allows images to be transmitted electronically.
- Electronic image transfer facilitates external quality assurance of the screening programme.
- Patients report that the lower flash intensity of digital camera systems is more comfortable.
- The review of images is popular with patients and carries potential for education. For the clinician it provides the means to monitor the disease over time.
- The proportion of unusable images is lower when mydriasis is used.
- Direct ophthalmoscopy, even with mydriasis, does not achieve the 80% sensitivity required for a screening test in the Diabetes UK (Exeter) Standards, regardless of the health care professional performing the test.
- Indirect ophthalmoscopy with mydriasis using a slit lamp has been shown to be sensitive and specific enough to be viable as a model for a national screening programme. Assessing the large number of people involved for quality assurance would be difficult. The method requires considerable skill and the critical size of the caseload, below which practitioners may be unable to maintain their skills, is uncertain.

- Ophthalmoscopy carries the disadvantage that there is no hard record for quality assurance or monitoring progressive changes.

Features of an acceptable national programme: an integrated pattern of care

The main features for any acceptable national programme are:

- Systematic call and recall of all eligible patients
- Trained professionals
- Recorded outcomes
- Targets and standards
- Quality assurance
- Promotion of uptake of screening
- Efficient and appropriate follow-up of all those with retinopathy.

Organisation of diabetic eye screening in primary care

Maintain a practice register of all people with diabetes. Check that the numbers match the expected prevalence in the locality.

When a person with diabetes is seen for review

- Ensure that the person understands the significance of diabetic eye disease and the need for an annual sight test (visual acuity) and eye examination, even though there may be no symptoms.
- Check that visual acuity and eye examinations have been performed within the last 12 months.
- Make sure patients are aware of the local eye screening programme and how to access it. Give him or her a leaflet explaining the scheme (see the example in Fig. 10.1).
- If visual acuity and eye examinations have not been performed, arrange for this to be done as soon as possible, either through the local eye screening scheme or refer to the local specialist diabetes service.
- If visual acuity and eye examinations have been performed, check the result and that appropriate action has been taken.
- Ensure that the recall and follow-up system is in place for the next annual sight test and eye screening to take place (see the example letter and form in Figs 10.2 and 10.3).

Why do I need my eyes screened?

Diabetic Retinopathy is a complication that can affect anyone who has diabetes, whether they are treated with insulin, tablets or diet.

Retinopathy generally has no obvious symptoms until it is well advanced. This is why an examination by an approved screener is so important.

Sheffield Diabetes Eye Screening Programme

هذا المنشور متوفر أيضا باللغة العربية والبنغالية والصينية والصومالية والأردية

یہ کتابچہ اردو، عربی، بنگال، چائنیز، اور صومالی زبانوں میں بھی دستیاب ہے۔

小冊另備阿拉伯文，孟加拉文，中文，索馬里文和身都文譯版。

Xaashidan waxaa la heli karaa iyadoo af Soomaali kuqoran

এই লিফলেটি আরবি, বাংলা, চাইনীজ, সোমালী এবং উর্দু ভাষাতে পাওয়া যাবে।

Sheffield Diabetes
Eye Screening
Programme

Johanne Wilson
Co-ordinator

Tel   0114 271 1821
Fax   0114 271 1931

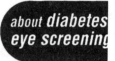

What is Retinopathy?

Retinopathy is the name given to changes in the blood vessels supplying the retina 'the seeing part of the eye'.

Blood vessels can become blocked, leaky or grow haphazardly. This then affects the way visual images are received by the retina and, if left untreated, can damage your vision.

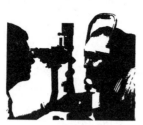

What does the screening involve?

The examination will involve a thorough check of the back of your eyes. To do this the optometrist will need to dilate your pupils in order for him/her to see the retina. This is done by using special eye drops which can sting at first, and can effect your vision for several hours. It is therefore important to:

- avoid driving to the appointment

- attend with someone if you are unsteady

- wear sun glasses if it is a bright day

How long will it take?

The examination will take approximately 40 minutes during this time your diabetes eye examination will be carried out and you will also be tested for glaucoma (raised eye pressure) which is easily treated.

What happens next?

If the optometrist feels you need a further examination he/she will then refer you to the Eye Department at the Royal Hallamshire Hospital.

If all is well you will be asked to see an optometrist again in 12 months time.

Queries?

If you have any questions about the screening, please do not hesitate to contact one of the optometrists on your list who will be happy to help or your GP.

Fig. 10.1 Example of a Local Diabetes Eye Screening Programme Leaflet (Sheffield)

Sheffield Diabetes Eye Screening Programme

Royal Hallamshire Hospital
Glossop Road
Sheffield S10 2JF

Tel: 0114 - 271 1821
Fax: 0114 - 271 1931

2 August 2001

Mrs P Johnston
The Tannery
Black Terrace
SHEFFIELD
S1 1XX

Dear Mrs Johnston

As part of your diabetes care, I would like to inform you that you are now due for a vision test and eye examination. Please follow the steps below:

1. Ensure that the details on the enclosed screening form are correct. If there are changes to be made, write them on the form. (There is no need to telephone the co-ordinator).

2. Telephone one of the opticians named on the list attached, and state that you have received your screening form and need to make an appointment. Please ensure that the appointment is made with the person whose name is on the list.

   Note: you DO NOT attend the hospital for this appointment

3. Take the enclosed screening form with you to your appointment and give it to the optician on arrival.

Please avoid driving to this appointment.

Please note: If you attend the Eye Department or Diabetes Centre at the Royal Hallamshire Hospital or the Diabetes Centre at the Northern General Hospital, please contact the Eye Screening Office on the above telephone number BEFORE you make your appointment with the optician.

If you have any further queries please contact the screening department.

Yours sincerely

J Smith
Co-ordinator

Fig. 10.2 Example of a Local Diabetes Eye Screening Programme Recall Letter (Sheffield)

Patient Information	Diabetes Data	GP Information
Our Ref. *123* NHS No. *22222* Surname *SMITH* Forename *MARGARET* Address *2 WHITE CLOSE* *SHEFFIELD* Postcode *S1002FT* DOB *25/12/48*	Duration Control: ~~DIET~~/TABLETS/INSULIN Care For Follow Up Of Diabetes Specify: GP/RHH/NGH/SCH/Other	Name *DR F. BLOGGS* Practice *ACORN MEDICAL PRACT.* *OAKTREE ROAD* Address *SHEFFIELD* Postcode *S1002FP* Previous Ophthal. Attend. Y /(N) Consultant

Examination Date: ....

	R	L	FUNDUS	R	L	ACTION	Tick
			Normal			Routine Recall	
Visual Acuity (Best Corrected)			Background DR			Routine Recall	
Previous Visual Acuity Date:			Preproliferative DR			Early Referral	
PINHOLE ACUITY			Vitreous Haemorrhage			Urgent Referral	
CORNEA			Proliferation			Urgent Referral	
IRIS			Retinal Detachment			Urgent Referral	
LENS			Mild Maculopathy			Routine Recall	
VITREOUS			Moderate Maculopathy			Routine Referral	
IOP (pneumo/applan)			Severe Maculopathy			Early Referral	
			Previous Laser RX	Y/N	Y/N		
			Other			Specify	

Any Pre-Existing Pathology: ....

Any other Information / Referral / Sketches:

Stamp

Examiner: ....   Signature: ....

CSUH Payment Slip   NHS No: *22222* ....

Patient: Surname: ....*SMITH*..............................   Forename *MARGARET* ....

Address: *2 WHITE CLOSE*
SHEFFIED S100 2FT

I have examined the above patient with a mydriatic and claim the agreed fee ☐

I have examined the above patient without a mydriatic for the following reasons ☐

GOC No: ....

Examiner:

Practice Address: ....

Address for Payment if Different ....

Stamp

Fig. 10.3 Example of a Local Diabetes Eye Screening Programme multi-copy form (Sheffield). The top white form is retained by the optometrist, the green copy is for the patient, the yellow or pink copy is returned to the Diabetes Eye Screening Coordinator or sent to the GP

When the eye screening result is known

If the result is normal:

- Record the result and confirm the next screening date
- Ensure that the person with diabetes is aware of the result.

If the result is abnormal:

- Ensure that the findings and implications are explained to the patient.
- Ensure an appropriate referral to ophthalmology **if indicated**.
- Ensure there is a general assessment of diabetes control and associated vascular risk factors and treat further as necessary.
- Refer to a specialist diabetes clinic as per your local arrangements.
- Confirm the next screening date as indicated.

Audit: annual review of recording of screening visits and referrals.

The role of the primary care team

It is important that all people with diabetes are aware of the importance of eye screening and know why and how to access their local eye screening programme.

- Ensure that they are aware of the significance of diabetes eye disease and the need for regular eye examination regardless of any absence of symptoms.
- Make sure that they are aware of the local eye screening programme and how to access it.
- Explain that the NHS pays for diabetes eye screening programmes and there will be no charge to them.
- Give them a leaflet explaining the local programme (example shown in Fig. 10.1).
- Encourage them to attend.
- Unless symptoms (of visual deterioration) are present, advise the patient not to have visual acuity tested for 2–3 months immediately after diagnosis, because the lens may be affected by changes in blood glucose levels.
- Check that they have attended, that the results are recorded and that referral/other action has been taken if indicated.
- Note when the next annual eye examination is due.

Visual acuity

- Visual acuity is a simple test indicating the acuteness of central vision for distance and near or reading vision.
- In the condition of diabetes, normal visual acuity may be shown, even though diabetic retinopathy is demonstrated by fundoscopy.
- The testing of visual acuity in people with diabetes is necessary because normal to good vision is required for the following reasons:
  - checking monitoring strips
  - checking tablets taken (type and dose)
  - checking insulin given (type, species and dose)
  - inspecting feet
  - checking skin lesions (for infection)
  - checking injection sites
  - reading instructions/educational material.
- Visual acuity should be checked annually and followed up by a fundoscopy examination through dilated pupils.
- If pupils are dilated before visual acuity is checked, the patient will be unable to see the test chart.
- If visual acuity has deteriorated and no diabetic retinopathy is detected by fundoscopy, the person with diabetes should be advised to visit an ophthalmic optician for optical tests and sight correction if required.
- Sight deterioration may be caused by a cataract which (if mature) requires referral to an ophthalmologist for removal (both eyes may be affected by cataracts).
- If diabetic retinopathy is detected and is sight threatening, urgent referral to an ophthalmologist is required.
- During stabilisation of diabetes (after diagnosis or where medication or insulin has been introduced or adjusted), visual disturbances, such as blurred vision, may be experienced. These visual changes may vary from individual to individual and will improve in time.
- Possible visual changes such as these should be explained (they occur as a result of changes in glucose levels in the lens of the eye).
- The person concerned should be reassured and told that, once blood glucose levels settle, vision will improve.
- On diagnosis and if alterations in therapy are made (such as a change from medication to insulin), the person concerned should be advised not to visit an optician until visual changes have settled (this may be a period of 2–3 months).
- Considerable inconvenience and expense (if new spectacles are advised) will be incurred by the person with diabetes if they are not correctly informed of the possibility of visual changes.

Note: annual eye tests (by an optician) are free for people with diabetes.

Opticians

There are three types of optician.

The dispensing optician

- The dispensing optician is available almost everywhere and can be found in many high streets.
- The dispensing optician tests sight, prescribes and provides spectacles according to the prescription.
- The dispensing optician does not detect other ophthalmic defects.

The contact lens fitter

- The contact lens fitter specialises in contact lens prescription and provision.
- The contact lens fitter tests sight, prescribes and provides contact lenses (and lens care advice/preparations).

Note: contact lenses can be used by people with diabetes. Soft contact lenses are generally advised.

The ophthalmic optician (optometrist)

- The ophthalmic optician is available almost everywhere.
- The ophthalmic optician tests sight, prescribes and provides spectacles according to the prescription.
- The ophthalmic optician can test for other eye problems, e.g. raised intraocular pressure (glaucoma).
- The ophthalmic optician can detect other defects, including diabetic retinopathy.
- Ophthalmic opticians are used by many general practitioners to screen for diabetic retinopathy. If retinopathy is detected by the optician a 'green card' with a record of the optician's examination is sent to the general practitioner, who then refers the patient to an ophthalmologist – if this is indicated.

Note: although experienced practitioners at ophthalmoscopy, ophthalmic opticians screening for diabetic retinopathy do not always dilate pupils before fundoscopy examination. Dilatation of the pupils (by instillation of mydriatic drops) is essential for the detection of diabetic retinopathy – particularly peripheral maculopathy (retinopathy detected at the periphery of the retinal fundus and not uncommon in people with type 2 diabetes of long duration; this may also be present at diagnosis).

Fundoscopy

Equipment

- A darkened room
- An approved ophthalmoscope with good batteries
- Mydriatic drops (tropicamide 0.5% or 1%). Tropicamide 1% may be necessary (particularly for people with dark-brown irises)
- Tissues.

Preparation of patient

- The patient should be pre-warned of fundoscopy examination and, if necessary, accompanied (particularly if elderly).
- Short distance vision is affected by the mydriatic drops (effect 2–4 hours), although blurring of vision may be experienced for up to 24 hours.
- Mydriatic drops do not preclude driving, although it may be prudent for the patient to avoid this.
- Mydriatic drops do not require reversal.
- Darkened glasses (sunglasses) should be worn (after mydriatic drops) in bright sunlight.

Before pupil dilatation and fundoscopy examination, the following history should be taken:

- General medical history
- Diabetes history (type, duration, treatment)
- History of eye problems (hereditary eye disease, cataracts, chronic glaucoma, etc.) and any eye surgery or treatment undergone or in progress
- Any visual symptoms experienced
- Visual acuity (unaided or with distance spectacles, with or without 'pinhole' card)
- Examination of both eyes (for cataract, iritis rubeosis).

!Warning!

- If the patient has a lens implant in place after a cataract extraction, mydriatic drops should not be used.
- Mydriatic drops can precipitate closed angle glaucoma in patients with shallow anterior chambers. The onset is rapid and painful. The eye becomes red with a hazy cornea and blurred vision. This is, however, very rare. Should it occur, immediate ophthalmic treatment is required.
- The possibility of precipitation of acute glaucoma should not preclude the use of mydriatic drops and fundoscopy examination, because this complication is so rare and, in the practice situation, can be quickly referred for treatment.
- It is important that the retinas are screened annually for diabetic retinopathy.

Cataracts

- Cataracts are more common in older people.
- Studies suggest that cataracts occur more often and at an earlier age in people with diabetes.
- It is important that cataracts are monitored and extracted as soon as appropriate when found in people with diabetes, so that vision and independence are restored.
- Screening for diabetic retinopathy is facilitated once cataracts have been removed.

Age-related macular degeneration

Age-related macular degeneration is a common cause of visual loss in older people. There is no effective treatment for this condition.

Chronic glaucoma

- Chronic glaucoma (as well as cataract) is more common in people with diabetes.
- The development of chronic glaucoma is slow and painless.
- It is important that intraocular pressure is measured and recorded annually.
- The measurement of intraocular pressure may be carried out in general practice (with appropriate equipment), by an ophthalmic optician or in screening programmes carried out by hospital ophthalmic departments.

- People with diabetes and individuals (aged 40 years and over) who are close relatives to known glaucoma patients are eligible for free NHS tests for the detection of glaucoma.
- Chronic glaucoma results in a gradual reduction in the peripheral field of vision so insidious that the patient is unaware, even at a late stage, when tunnel vision develops.
- Treatment consists of eye drops or oral agents. If these fail, surgical trabeculectomy or laser therapy is carried out.

Fundoscopy examination – step by step

Instilling mydriatic drops

- Explain procedure to patient.
- Warn patient that drops will sting for a few moments.
- Sit patient in chair with head back.
- Stand behind patient and ask him or her to look up.
- Pull down lower eyelid and allow drop to fall into lower fornix.
- The eye will close in a reflex action.
- Mop with tissues.
- Repeat in other eye.
- Keep patient seated in darkened room for 15–20 minutes (to allow pupils to dilate as fully as possible).
- If pupils do not dilate sufficiently after the above procedure, a further drop in each eye may be necessary.

After fundoscopy examination by doctor

- Record results
- Check vision is satisfactory (this may be blurred)
- Check transport/availability of accompanying person (particularly if patient is elderly) before allowing home.

If diabetic retinopathy is detected

- The patient should be informed.
- Information should be given as to the extent of retinal damage.
- If the retinopathy is sight threatening, immediate referral should be made to an ophthalmologist.
- A great deal of reassurance and support is required because of the fear surrounding possible visual loss and the fear of eye treatment (laser therapy or surgery).

Fig. 10.4 Laser therapy: patient information sheet

- The laser is a machine that produces a small spot of very bright light.
- The light is so bright it produces a burn wherever it is focused.
- The lasers used produce blue–green or occasionally red light.
- Although the laser makes a burn in your eye, it is not usually painful because the back of your eye (the retina) cannot feel pain.
- Sometimes, however, if you have had a lot of laser treatment, it may be painful and you will be offered a local anaesthetic.
- Laser treatment is almost always done in an outpatient department.
- You will be perfectly fit to go home after the treatment.
- Your vision may be blurred or you may be dazzled by bright light (take dark glasses with you).
- You should not drive home afterwards.
- It is best to be accompanied to the laser clinic.
- After the treatment, you may notice some reduction in your sight. This usually only lasts a short time and only occasionally as much as a week. Occasionally you may experience headaches.
- As only one eye is treated at a time, if your other eye sees well, your vision should not be too badly affected.
- Most people do not need to take time off work after treatment.
- If you declare on your driving licence application form that you have had laser treatment, as you are required to do, it is likely that you will have to have a visual fields test (to test the extent of your vision).
- If you have to have large amounts of laser treatment, your field of vision may be affected.
- Provided that you can read a number plate at 25 metres (80 feet) with or without spectacles, and you pass the visual fields test, as most people do, there will be no problem about you driving.

- Detailed explanations regarding the degree of retinal damage (after possible further tests – such as retinal photography) and a plan of treatment will be given by the ophthalmologist.
- Information regarding laser therapy for patients is provided (Fig. 10.4).

Further reading

Alexander WD (1998). *Diabetic Retinopathy: A guide for diabetes care teams.* Oxford: Blackwell Science Ltd.

Ariffin A, Hill RD, Leigh O (1992). *Diabetes and Primary Eye Care.* Oxford: Blackwell Science Publications.

Diabetes UK (2000). *Advisory Panel Final Report to the UK National Screening Committee.* London: Diabetes UK (website: www.diabetic-retinopathy. screening.nhs.uk/recommendations.html).

11 Foot care and surveillance

■ Foot care
■ Feet at risk
■ Treatment

At annual review and if identified as 'at risk' more frequently, the primary care team should be concerned with foot care as an essential part of diabetes care and surveillance.

There are difficulties in foot education, i.e. patients can have difficulties taking messages on board when they cannot feel the damage that is being done. In addition, patients at risk need specifically to be made aware if they have existing neuropathy and ischaemia, and what that means to them.

Clinical guidelines for type 2 diabetes: prevention and management of foot problems

(This guideline does not deal with the management of risk factors such as raised blood glucose levels, smoking, raised lipid levels, raised blood pressure.) Based on graded evidence, national collaborative guidelines (2000, for review in 2003) are available.

Principal recommendations

Foot care for all people with diabetes
■ Arrange recall and annual review of complications and their risk factors by trained personnel.
■ Examine feet and lower legs, as part of annual review to detect risk factors for ulceration.
■ Include:
  ◆ testing of foot sensation using a 10-g monofilament or vibration
  ◆ palpation of foot pulses
  ◆ inspection of foot shape and footwear.

Classify foot risk as: **low current risk** or **at risk** or **high risk** or **ulcerated foot**.

Foot care for the *low current risk* foot (normal sensation, palpable pulses)
■ Agree a management plan including foot care education with each person.

Foot care for the *at risk* foot (neuropathy or absent pulses or other risk factor)
■ If previous foot ulcer or deformity or skin changes manage as *high risk*
■ Enhance foot care education
■ Inspect feet 3- to 6-monthly
■ Advise on appropriate footwear
■ Review need for vascular assessment.

Foot care for the *high risk* foot (risk factor + deformity or skin changes or previous ulcer)
■ Arrange frequent review (1- to 3-monthly) from specialised podiatry/foot care team.
■ At each regular diabetes review, evaluate the provision of:
  ◆ intensified foot care education
  ◆ specialist footwear and insoles
  ◆ frequent (according to need) skin and nail care.
■ Review education/footwear/vascular status as for the *at risk* foot.
■ Ensure special arrangements for those people with disabilities or immobility.

Foot care for the *ulcerated* foot
■ Arrange, urgently, foot ulcer care from a team with specialist expertise.
■ Expect that team to ensure as a minimum:
  ◆ investigation and treatment of vascular insufficiency
  ◆ local wound management, appropriate dressings and débridement as indicated
  ◆ systemic antibiotic therapy for cellulitis or bone infection
  ◆ effective means of distributing foot pressures, e.g. specialist footwear, casts
  ◆ tight blood glucose control.

Foot care emergency: new ulceration, cellulitis, discoloration
Referral to specialised podiatry/foot care team.

Foot care

Foot care for people with diabetes attending the hospital

A member of the primary care team should check annually (from people with diabetes attending the surgery or from hospital letters held in the general practice records) for the following:

- That feet have been examined.
- That shoes have been examined.
- That action has been taken (if appropriate) following the detection of foot problems or inappropriate footwear.
- That education about foot care and shoes has been provided.

Foot care for people with diabetes attending the practice

Foot care for people with diabetes attending the practice should be provided for the following:

- People with diabetes solely attending the practice for their care.
- People attending the practice where care is 'integrated/shared' and foot care has not been provided by the hospital.
- People who are housebound and cannot attend hospital or practice for foot care.

What foot care should be provided by the primary care team?

- Identification of people with diabetes 'at risk' of foot problems.
- An annual examination of both feet (more often for those 'at risk').
- An annual examination of shoes.
- Education about foot care and footwear.
- Appropriate and timely referral for chiropody (podiatry) treatment.
- Appropriate and timely referral to a specialist foot clinic (if needed).

Feet at risk

The non-diabetic foot

It should be remembered that feet are at risk in the non-diabetic population under the following conditions.

The young person

- Ill-fitting footwear
- Poor quality footwear
- Trauma
- Congenital spine, hip, lower limb deformities
- In pregnant women – changing weight and gait.

In middle age

- Foot deformities
- Ill-fitting footwear
- Poor quality footwear
- Increasing weight
- Changing gait.

Elderly people

- Poor vision
- Decreasing mobility
- Living alone
- Foot deformities
- Poor circulation
- Concurrent medical problems
- Ill-fitting footwear
- Poor quality footwear
- Changing weight
- Changing gait.

The diabetic foot

The two major complications of diabetes, causing foot ulceration, are (Fig. 11.1):

- Abnormal circulation (micro- and macrovascular disease – ischaemia)
- Diabetic neuropathy (autonomic and peripheral).

It is important to recognise that one or other or both of these complications may be present in the same patient and to be able to recognise the differences between them and the associated factors leading to foot ulceration.

Fig. 11.1 The major complications of diabetes causing foot problems

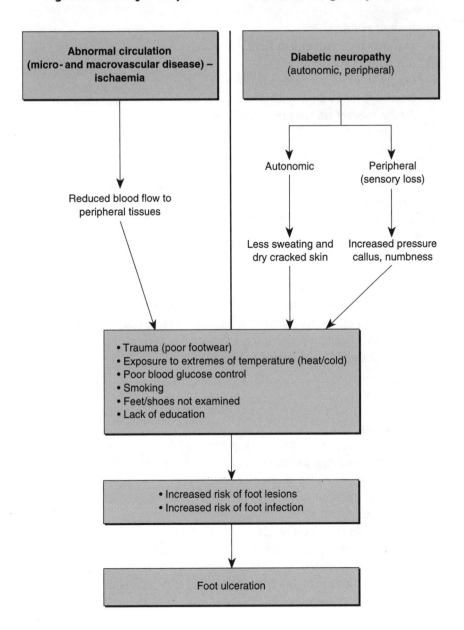

Examination of the feet

Equipment required

- Examination couch or foot stool (second chair)
- A good light source
- Cotton wool (to test 'light' sensation)
- Neurotips (or 10 g monofilament may be used – for 'sharp' sensation)
- Patella hammer (to test knee/ankle jerk)
- A 'C' tuning fork CO128 (to test vibration perception)
- Wound swab (accompanying laboratory form).

Note: Doppler ultrasound can be used for the measurement of blood flow and a biothesiometer can be used for the detection of diminished vibration perception. These two items of equipment are expensive and not essential.

The examination

- Shoes, socks (tights or stockings) should be removed.
- The patient should be examined lying on a couch or seated comfortably with both legs and feet raised (on a foot stool or second chair).
- Both feet should be examined for the following:
  - condition of the skin (lower legs and feet)
  - check for dry, flaky skin
  - check for cracks or evidence of fungal infection between each toe (athlete's foot)
  - check colour of skin (lower legs and feet)
  - check for corns, calluses other deformities (particularly on pressure-bearing points, e.g. metatarsal heads)
  - check condition of toe nails (whether thickened, long or horny)
  - check nail-cutting technique/ingrowing toe nails
  - check for discoloration/abnormal skin lesions
  - check for evidence of infection, i.e. pain, lack of pain, numbness, inflammation, cellulitis or exudate (which may be purulent)
  - ensure that upper, lower surfaces of feet and toes (including heels) are carefully examined.
- All abnormalities/changes should be recorded.
- A doctor or further trained member of the primary care team should complete the examination of the feet for the following:
  - palpation of dorsalis pedis and posterior tibial pulses
  - if ischaemia is severe, pulses throughout the lower limb should be palpated
  - changed, diminished or absent pulses should be recorded

Table 11.1 The ischaemic and neuropathic foot

The ischaemic foot	The neuropathic foot
History	**History**
Presence of intermittent claudication (calf pain) present when walking, relieved by rest	Corns, calluses and ulcers are usually painful
Rest pain is a constant severe pain in toes, foot or calf, even thighs and buttocks, when severe	Questioning may reveal that the patient is unaware of lesions or that they are not troublesome
Pain occurs at rest and is aggravated when in sleeping position	Enquire about general sensation (feeling in the legs and feet)
	A lack of feeling or 'pins and needles' or burning may be reported
Examination	**Examination**
Colour: pale to cyanosed	Colour: normal to pink
Temperature: cold	Temperature: warm
Pulses (dorsalis pedis posterior tibial): diminished or absent	Pulses (dorsalis pedis posterior tibial): present or may be full and bounding
Sensation: present	Sensation: diminished or absent
Knee/ankle jerk: present	Knee/ankle jerk: diminished or absent

- sensation testing – by checking light touch sensation, sharp/blunt discrimination and vibration perception
- testing for light touch, sharp/blunt discrimination and vibration perception should be carried out from toe to mid-calf region
- for comparison, the stimulus should first be applied to the patient's outstretched hand and then repeated on the lower limbs and feet – with the eyes closed
- testing for motor neuropathy should include examination for weakness or deformities in the toes and feet

- in addition, knee and ankle jerks should be checked (with a patella/tendon hammer)
- sensation defects should be recorded
- foot ulcers should be examined for inflammation and discharge (and a swab taken for bacterial analysis)
- foot problems identified should be recorded and discussed with the patient as appropriate.

Examination of the shoes

Shoes should be examined inside and outside for:

- Evidence of wear and tear generally
- The need for repair
- Evidence of gait change (one shoe more worn than the other)
- Evidence of excessive weight bearing (heel on sole worn down)
- Evidence of perforation of soles or heels (by nails, etc.)
- Evidence of abrasive heels (especially with new shoes)
- Evidence of damaging projections inside the shoes (causing pressure)
- Evidence of worn insoles (causing pressure)
- Problems identified with shoes should be recorded and discussed with the patient.

Examination of socks/tights/stockings

Socks, tight or stocking should be examined for:

- Type of material (whether constricting – nylon or elasticated)
- Type of washing powder used (biological washing powders can be irritant)
- Method of holding up (e.g. garters should not be used)
- Presence and thickness of seams (these can cause traumatic ulcers)
- Problems identified should be recorded and discussed with the patient.

Identification of people at risk of diabetic foot problems

People with diabetes 'at risk' of foot problems should be identified and recorded on the diabetes register, and/or on the recall system – for more frequent follow-up.

Those at risk are:

- People with peripheral vascular disease (ischaemia)
- People with neuropathy

- Elderly people
- People with poor vision
- People unable to care for their own feet
- People living alone
- People with poor mobility/dexterity
- People with foot deformities
- People with a history of foot ulceration
- People who are heavy smokers
- People with poor glycaemic control.

Fig. 11.2 Foot

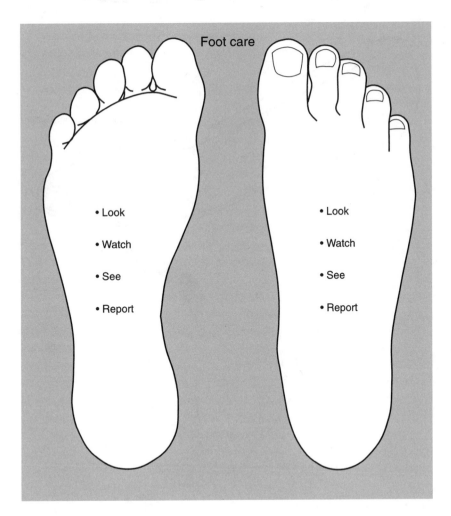

Foot care

- Look
- Watch
- See
- Report

- Look
- Watch
- See
- Report

Fig. 11.3 Shoes

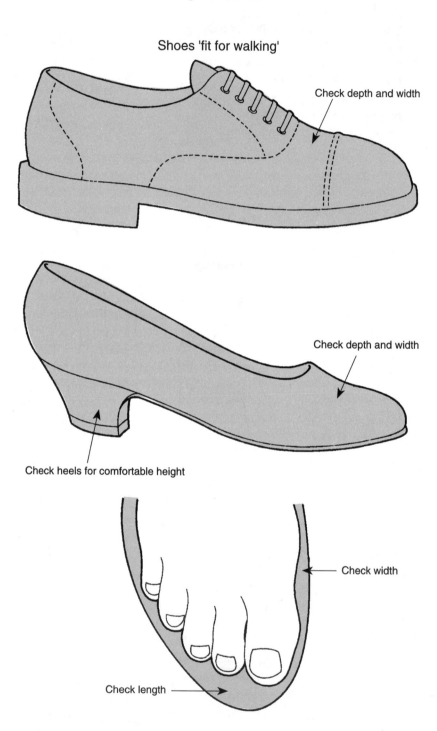

Shoes 'fit for walking'

Check depth and width

Check depth and width

Check heels for comfortable height

Check width

Check length

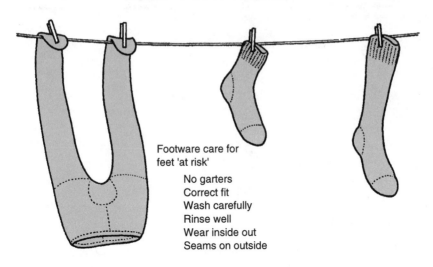

Fig. 11.4 Socks/stockings/tights

Footware care for
feet 'at risk'

No garters
Correct fit
Wash carefully
Rinse well
Wear inside out
Seams on outside

Treatment

Foot care advice

- Advice about foot care should be individually given and reinforced as and when appropriate (at least annually).
- Foot care advice should preferably be provided for the relative/carer, as the person with diabetes (particularly if they are 'at risk') may be unable to follow the advice themselves.
- An individual leaflet may be supplied, written in the presence of the person with diabetes, relative or carer.
- Foot care information leaflets may be available locally or free from Diabetes UK or pharmaceutical companies (see resources list, Appendix VIII).
- Information and advice for patients about foot care, shoes and footwear (socks, stockings, tights) are given in Tables 11.2, 11.3 and 11.4.

Table 11.2 Patient information: diabetes foot care advice: 10 points

- Inspect feet daily (if possible – use a mirror if you cannot reach your feet)

- Keep feet clean (wash well, dry between toes)

- Avoid extremes of temperature – heat/cold

- Avoid very hot baths (put cold water in first then add hot water; test with elbow)

- Avoid hot fires/radiators

- Avoid hot water bottles (use an electric heat pad and check safety annually or alternatively wear warm bed socks)

- Report sores, skin damage **immediately** to your doctor

- Cut nails according to shape of toe

- If you cannot cut nails – go to a State-Registered Chiropodist (podiatrist)

- Do not treat corns or calluses yourself – go to a State-Registered Chiropodist (podiatrist)

- Do not use surgical blades or corn-paring knives on your feet

- Keep skin moist (use hand cream, olive oil or E45 cream, available on prescription)

- Wear shoes or slippers at all times

Table 11.3 Patient information: diabetes care shoe advice: 10 points

■ Feel inside and check the outside of your shoes before putting them on (check for ridges, sharp points or protruding nails)

■ Buy shoes that fit well (depth, width and length, heels not too high – approximately 3–7 cm (1–2"))

■ Go to a shoe shop that will measure and fit your shoes correctly

■ Remember that shoes should be fitted individually (each foot is slightly different in shape and size)

■ If the shape of your foot has altered you may need specially fitted insoles or shoes (these can be supplied by your chiropodist [podiatrist] or shoe fitter)

■ Do not wear new shoes for long (no more than 1–2 hours at a time)

■ Newly fitted shoes should be slightly longer than your longest toe when you are standing – your foot lengthens when you walk (your toes should move freely inside your shoes)

■ Make sure shoes are not too tight (watch out for creases when you walk)

■ Make sure shoes are not too loose (watch out for your feet sliding or heels/toes rubbing)

■ Do not wear rubber boots for too long. Do not wear 'work' boots for too long (change into shoes as soon as you can)

11

Table 11.4 Patient information: diabetes care – footwear advice (socks, stockings, tights): 8 points

■ If possible, change socks, stockings or tights daily

■ Wear the correct size

■ Socks should be of natural fibres (wool or cotton) and loose fitting

■ Do not wear garters

■ Wash in non-irritant detergent (e.g. non-biological washing powder) and rinse well

■ If you have poor circulation or nerve damage, wear socks, stockings or tights inside out (so that the seams are on the outside of your foot)

■ Repair damaged socks, stockings, tights or discard and use new ones

■ If you have varicose veins, requiring support stockings – seek medical advice (for the correct type and size of stocking when you obtain your prescription)

Treatment of diabetic foot ulcers by the primary care team

If foot ulcers are reported to, or detected by, the primary care team, the following procedure should be carried out:

■ Both feet should be examined
■ Glycaemic control should be reviewed
■ A wound swab should be taken (if appropriate)
■ If infection is present, antibiotics should be prescribed (these may be required long term)
■ The foot and lower limb should be rested whenever possible
■ When resting – the foot and lower limb should be elevated (at least to hip level)
■ Light non-adherent dressings should be used
■ Elastoplast should be used on the skin with great care and only when essential
■ Constricting (elastic) bandages should not be used

- Both feet should be examined regularly
- If infection persists, the ulcer does not heal or glycaemic control is poor, referral to a diabetes foot clinic (or the hospital diabetes team) should be made.

Criteria for referral to specialist foot clinic or hospital diabetes team

Referral should be made for the following reasons:

- The presence of a non-healing foot ulcer
- Severe ischaemia
- Autonomic or peripheral neuropathy causing sensory loss
- Pain/numbness in feet or lower limbs
- Poor 'glycaemic' control in those identified 'at risk' of foot problems
- Those with a history of foot ulceration
- People with a foot deformity (which may be caused by neuropathy)
- Where osteomyelitis is suspected (an X-ray is required to confirm this)
- People requiring 'custom-made' insoles or special shoes
- People identified 'at risk' requiring regular chiropody (podiatry) and surveillance (outside the scope of the primary care team).

Criteria for referral to a State-Registered Chiropodist (podiatrist)

Referral should be made for the following reasons:

- Where toe nails cannot be cut by the person with diabetes (as a result of visual impairment, etc.)
- Where toe nails cannot be cut by the relative or carer
- Where corns or calluses require treatment
- Where insoles or special shoes may be required
- Where general foot care/footwear advice is needed
- Where urgent chiropodist (podiatrist) treatment is required
- Where an assessment is needed
- Where regular surveillance is required.

Further reading

British Diabetic Association (1993). Non-insulin-dependent diabetes. *Balance for Beginners* 44–6.

Edmonds ME, Foster AVM (2000). *Managing the Diabetic Foot*. Oxford: Blackwell Science.

Hutchinson A, McIntosh A, Feder G, Home PD, Young R (2000). *Clinical Guidelines for Type 2 Diabetes: Prevention and management of foot problems*. London: Royal College of General Practitioners

Woodburn J, Thomson C (1991). The diabetic foot 1991. *Diabetic Nursing* **2**(2): 3–5.

12 Aspects of culture relating to diabetes care

- Cultural sensitivities and diabetes care
- Prevalence and complications
- Cultural locking or barriers
- Cultures/Customs
- Etiquette in examination
- Hinduism
- Islam
- Sikhism
- Judaism
- African–Caribbean
- Hot and cold foods
- Food modification and dietary advice

Living with diabetes involves all aspects of life at any age and an understanding of culture is helpful in order to avoid giving inappropriate advice, causing misunderstandings or even giving offence.

- Religion and culture can vary greatly even within limited geographical areas.
- It is important to recognise family, social, local and country-wide religions and cultural customs.
- Religious and cultural customs may change as people move from one stage of life to another (e.g. the child coming of age).
- Sex is of importance in many cultures.
- Hierarchy in a household may also be significant.
- Holy days or holidays involve a change in lifestyle for a period of time.
- Food is of great importance in all societies, and the culture and customs surrounding it may be based on religious beliefs and should be respected accordingly.
- Religion may form the basis of the daily routine of prayers, work, relaxation and meal times.
- Certain foods (e.g. pork or beef) may be prohibited in some religions.
- Followers of religions may choose a devout and conservative path, whereas others may have a more relaxed view of the rules.

- Personal conscience dictates the choice of the individual about which route they will follow.
- Cultural preconceptions should be avoided if possible.
- Understanding and respect for each individual is required.

Cultural sensitivities and diabetes care

Many people have migrated from all the continents of the world at various periods in British history, as the British have also emigrated to all parts of the world. The movements of people from Asian and African–Caribbean subcontinents have brought people whose most valuable possessions are their cultural heritage, native customs, religion and languages.

People from a south Asian background came from two different subcontinents: the first generation of migrants came directly from the Asian subcontinent, and the second generation first migrated to the African subcontinents and then came to live in UK after such events as the Ugandan crisis. Although both generations of south Asian migrants had their own cultural enrichments, there is a vast difference in the perception of health care of the two. Migrants from Asian subcontinents maintained the native culture of health care, with its traditional ethos and health beliefs to this day, whereas those from the Caribbean were influenced by Western culture and traditions, adopting the changing culture of health care with open minds, even though some of them still maintained traditional health beliefs.

As living with diabetes involves all aspects of life at any age, it is prudent for health care workers to have an understanding of the sensitive cultural issues before approaching or providing care to people of different ethnic origins to avoid giving inappropriate advice or causing misunderstanding which could lead to poor reception of, and adherence to, care management.

Prevalence and complications

In 1997 the worldwide incidence of diabetes was 2.1%. It is expected that, by 2010, the incidence will increase 3%, with 61% of people with diabetes living in Asia. Studies in Southall (west London) and Coventry have shown two- to fivefold increases of diabetes in Indo-Asians from the Indian subcontinent and their descendants. Professor George Alberti, in 1999, gave an overview reflecting on the prevalence of diabetes in Indo-Asian people, which varied from 1.2% to 16%, with considerable rural and urban variation as a result of changing lifestyles.

The diabetes appears to develop at a relatively younger age in Asian people and therefore it is more likely that the prevalence and complications will increase with advancing age and socioeconomic status.

The prevalence of complications is similar to that of white people, although death from coronary artery disease and the incidence of end-stage renal failure are higher in Indo-Asians. The reasons for poor outcomes have been identified as poor glycaemic control and poor knowledge of diabetes in Indo-Asians, and underlying environmental, genetic predisposition and cultural influences contribute to this situation.

Cultural locking or barriers

The migrants from the first and second generations maintain their culture and traditional views more strongly than the third generation.

Communication

There are more than one billion people currently living in south Asia (i.e. the Indian subcontinent). India is the most populated country in the world after China, and Pakistan and Bangladesh are also in the top ten. In all the capital cities of south Asia an Indo-Aryan language, which is the most eastern group of the Indo-European family, is predominant: Hindi in Delhi, Urdu and Punjabi in Islamabad, Bangali in Dhaka, Sinhalese in Colombo and Nepali in Kathmandu. Communication remains one of the major barriers among these native migrants. Fortunately, all these migrants are from the old or new commonwealth where English remains the second language in the country of origin. Medicine and law are still practised in English in most of the commonwealth countries. Therefore they are used to having interpreters. Although it is necessary to have an interpreter for health officials or patients, family members or advocates provide a more acceptable approach to native migrants.

People from ethnic minorities shouldn't be expected to speak English well. With a little extra effort and patience communication can be fruitful. English, although having undergone modifications over almost four centuries of use in south Asia, still plays an important role in all the countries of south Asia and is widely spoken in towns and cities by the third generation. Link workers and telephone translation services are available in many health authorities for use in communicating with immigrant patients from other countries who have little knowledge of English. Enquire at your Health Authority (health education promotion) and through community and social services.

12

Cultures/Customs

Problems can arise when doctors or nurses of one culture are dealing with patients who are migrants from other cultures. It is not possible to describe all the cultures represented in the UK, but some explanations of aspects that could give rise to health hazards is necessary to avoid diagnostic or management traps. Individuals are often expected to behave in a prescribed fashion in different cultures, and doctors/nurses may see patients from different cultures indulging in some of the habits described in the following.

Betel chewing

Betel is an after-dinner delicacy used by adult Asians and Malaysians. According to the *Encyclopaedia Britannia*, a quarter of the world's population practises this habit. Betel leaf is used as a raper; it contains betel nut, limestone paste, catechu, cardamom, rose hips, turmeric root, silver foil and tobacco. Betel leaf, cardamom and rosehips are carminatives – a source of vitamin C – and have a pleasant odour. Betel nut, catechu and lime paste are rich sources of calcium and iron, preventing deficiencies. Patients with diabetes from such ethnic backgrounds commonly use betel; if limited in its use, it serves a healthy purpose, but excessive use can predispose to gallstones, and kidney and bladder stones. Lime paste predisposes to chronic buccal ulceration and the tobacco chewed in betal leaf has carcinogenic properties. It is important to be aware of these when caring for patients with diabetes from these backgrounds.

Hooka smoking

Doctors/nurses should be aware that this is a common practice and social custom among adult Asian men and women (particularly Muslim and Bangladeshi). The hooka is a smoking apparatus that consists of a flask filled with water, with two tubes attached. One tube is topped by a funnel containing lighted coals, beneath which is a metal lid over a layer of tobacco leaves or paste; the second tube has one end under the water in the flask and the other is fitted with a mouthpiece. Tobacco vapour filtered through the water is inhaled through the mouthpiece.

Cigarette and beedi smoking

This is a quite common among Hindus, Muslims and Bangladeshis even in the first and second generations. There are 'cigarette shops' in various parts of the country where it can be bought. Beedi is rolled tobacco in a tobacco leaf and is commonly available in the Asian grocery shops as well as these 'cigarette shops'. Beedi has a very high tar content. People of Asian backgrounds commonly go for a walk after the evening meal to these 'cigarette shops', which are more of a social meeting place analogous to pubs in the indigenous culture of Britain.

Enquiries should be made of Asian patients with diabetes about their smoking and tobacco consumption habits, in view of the high incidence of coronary heart disease and large vessel disease among Asians.

Sarsoon oil (mustard oil)

In the Asian subcontinent, prolonged exposure to sunshine causes dryness of the skin. It is customary to apply sarsoon oil all over the body to counteract this. The oil is cheap, readily available in this country and very effective with a distinctive smell. Patients with diabetes could be advised to choose more readily available moisturising creams for the body.

Toilet and bathing habits

Asian, African or Chinese patients may take showers rather than baths because they have been brought up not to sit in the bathwater. Therefore it may not be acceptable to advise patients with diabetes from ethnic minorities to have a bath.

Most south Asians are accustomed to lavatories with a low seat, and washing with plenty of water instead of using paper for cleaning. Many people find it difficult to become accustomed to Western practice. Western men prefer to stand for urination, whereas south Asian men prefer to sit.

Extended family systems are still the norm among south Asian migrants to the UK, although, among the third generation, some live in single units under the influence of the indigenous culture. In the extended family, the mother-in-law plays a major role in cooking and shopping for the whole family. Many south Asians living in this country have, however, adapted their lifestyle to the environment, incorporating many Western features of food, meal habits and change in activity level (often taking less exercise than previously).

Alcohol

Alcohol is commonly consumed and abused by many south Asians although it is prohibited in some religions. It is often excessively consumed among professional and upper middle-class women/men.

It is important to ask Asian patients with diabetes about alcohol consumption.

Religion

It is impossible to write briefly about the religions in south Asia without fear of oversimplification. There are over 680 million Hindus in south Asia today, making them the largest single group.

The first Christians arrived within 60 years of the birth of Christ, and were influential in south India, particularly Kerala. Today there are about 18 million Christians in India, with a far smaller number in the other countries of south Asia.

The religious development did not stop with the arrival of Islam. A more recent religious reform movement in India that has made a significant impact is that of the Sikhs. Although numerically smaller than the Christian population, the Sikhs outnumber Jains and Buddhists and play a more major role in national life than any of the other minor religions.

The following are the commonly practised religions in south Asia:

- Hinduism, Jainism, Buddhism are commonly practised by Hindus.
- Islam is practised by Muslims.
- Sikhism is practised by Sikhs.
- Christianity is practised by Christians.
- Judaism is practised by Jews.
- Zoroastrianism is practised by Parsis or Persians.

The extended family system has always been the major strength in developing the culture of family members towards religious beliefs. One religious heritage that is commonly visible in any Asian house is the presence of a protected prayer place, whatever the Asian religion practised in the family.

Etiquette in examination

Greetings

The English have a personality profile of 'vision, hearing, touch'. African–Caribbeans, Asians, Chinese, east Europeans and even Americans have a personality profile of 'touch, hearing, vision'.

Manners

Examples of English manners include constant eye contact, speaking out loud, holding a conversation, standing at ease with a confident smile, listening without speaking and also being at ease with silence.

It is the opposite in Eastern cultures. You may well notice poor eye contact and the husband taking control of the conversation for the whole family.

History taking

In an African–Asian culture, the patient expects the doctor/nurse to know the diagnosis of the patient's problem without being questioned or examined because alternative medical practitioners used to make good guesses at their chronic condition without this.

Moreover there is more emphasis on physical symptoms than psychological ones, and patients expect a prescription rather than mere advice. Often they also would expect to have paid for drugs in their native land but not for the consultation.

British patients are only too happy to give their life and family history to the doctor/nurse, but African–Asian patients resist answering this line of questioning and view it with grave suspicion. The word 'I' is never used by African–Asian patients; 'please' and 'the' may not exist in their language. Their politeness is conveyed by gesture.

British people believe in the basic rights of privacy and free speech; they dislike personal questions being asked in public, and anyone using an aggressive approach or giving a verdict before a trial. In Eastern cultures these things are taken very lightly.

Examination

African–Asian women would prefer to be examined by a woman doctor, and men would be very embarrassed to be examined by a woman doctor. This may be misinterpreted by a health professional as sexual discrimination. Rectal examinations, enemas or giving suppositories, and referral to psychiatrists are all taboo in Eastern cultures.

It is well worth while, after having taken a detailed history and examination, to spend a few moments educating the patients about the British system of supportive counselling as well as drug therapy.

Hinduism

There are many different strands in Hinduism, and some Hindu scholars and philosophers talk of it as a religious and cultural tradition, in which the enormous variety of believes and practice can ultimately be interpreted as interwoven in a common view of the world. There are spiritual leaders and philosophers who are widely revered and there is an enormous range of literature that is treated as sacred. These are called Vedas and regarded as sacred by most Hindus. Not all Hindu groups believe in a single supreme God and, even today, there are adherents of several of the major systems of philosophy, which developed in the course of Hinduism. Hinduism activities range from everyday family life to great temple rituals. Hindu philosophy and practice have also affected many of those who belong to other religious traditions, particularly in terms of social institutions such as caste.

Beliefs

It is impossible to tie Hindu beliefs down to a universally accepted creed, although a number of ideas do run through intellectual and popular Hinduism. A former President of India, S. Radhakrishnan, described Hinduism as a power not an idea, not an intellectual proposition but a life conviction. Religion is consciousness of ultimate reality, not a theory about God.

Many Hindus accept that there are four major human goals: material prosperity (*Artha*), the satisfaction of desire (*Kama*), performing the duties laid down according to your position (*Dharma*), and achieving liberation from the endless cycle of re-births into which every one is locked (*Moksha*). It is to the last – the search for liberation – that the major school of Indian philosophy has devoted most attention.

Customs

It is common practice to have a picture of God or even a separate prayer place or temple in the house. Every member of the family takes a shower or bath in the morning and prays before leaving the house for daily tasks. It is common for them to offer sweets and dry or fresh fruit to God during their prayers. These are consumed by the family members on a daily basis.

Social class

As with the word Hinduism itself, caste was not an indigenous term. It was applied by the Portuguese to the dominant social institution that they found practised on their arrival in India. A person is born into his or her caste – society is divided into different levels, linked to traditional occupations and to each person's duty in society.

There are five main castes and within each caste there are many subcastes in India:

1. Brahmins: are the priestly Varna believed to be the upper caste.
2. Kshatryas (Rajput): are the warrior Varna.
3. Vaishyas: the trading community.
4. Sudras: they are classified as agriculturists or farmers.
5. Untouchables: the outcast who were left behind to do impure jobs and associated with dealing with the dead or with excrement.

Although these caste systems are still practised in India, migrants have adopted more open views. Most marriages are still encouraged within their own castes. Asian migrants from African–Caribbean continents are more orthodox and strict with the caste system even in this country.

Festivals

There are three important festivals celebrated by many Hindus:

- *Holi:* a festival of colour welcoming the arrival of spring with colours (February/March).
- *Deshara:* a festival celebrating the death of Demon Rawana (mostly October).
- *Dewali:* a festival of light, joy and sharing (October/November). It is similar to Christmas. People celebrate the return of Lord Ramma after killing the Demon Rawana. It follows the start of the New Year for the trading community.

All the above festivals have one thing in common: the exchange of sweets/dry fruit or other sweet items. People visit each other and share sweets and rich fried food. Most people with diabetes find it very difficult to refuse these sweet-meats and end up with hyperglycaemia or taking extra oral hypoglycaemic agents without informing their doctor/nurse. Many Asian people still feel very strongly stigmatised with a diagnosis of diabetes. It is still considered as a contagious disease and people with diabetes find it difficult to arrange marriages for their children.

Buddhism and Jainism are practised mostly by Hindus in south Asia, although they are practised in only the northern part of India with some influence in the southern parts. Both religions travelled widely to Burma, Thailand, Malaysia and other Far Eastern countries, more or less following Hindu culture and customs. They are more open minded about their marriages and follow Lord Buddha and Saint Mahavir.

Food

On the whole Hindus (Buddhist and Jains) are vegetarian, although sweets are consumed more or less daily. Rich fried food is consumed at celebrations and festivities; cows are sacred to orthodox Hindus and prayed to, so beef is not eaten by Hindus. Many women fast for one or two days in a week or on certain festive occasions. They may consume fruits, sweets or milk puddings. Full cream milk is commonly used for puddings, etc.

Islam

Muslims are a highly visible community in all the countries of south Asia today. Islam is a faith of the overwhelming majority of people in Pakistan and Bangladesh. Its influence stretches beyond the present distribution of 'Muslim states'. India alone has over 100 million Muslims and is one of the largest Muslim populations in the world. Even Nepal and Sri Lanka, predominantly Hindu and Buddhist, have significant Muslim communities.

Muslims have two sects: Sunni and Shi'Is. They were split in the early centuries on political and religious grounds. Both groups' sects venerate Qur'an but have different Hadis. They also have different views about Mohammed the prophet and his Successor.

Islam has no priesthood; the authority of the Imams derives from social customs and their authority to interpret the scripture rather than from defined status.

Beliefs

Unlike Hinduism, Islam has a fundamental creed. There is no God but God, and Mohammed is the prophet of God *(La-illha- illa'uh Mohammed Rasulu'llah)*.

Qu'ran is the supreme authority on Islam teaching and faith, which preaches the belief in body resurrection after death and in the reality of Heaven and Hell. It lays down social rules and religious behaviours. Islam also prohibits any distinction on the basis of race and colour, and there is a strong antipathy to the representation of the human figure.

There are five obligatory requirements imposed on Muslims:

1. Daily prayers are performed at daybreak, noon, afternoon, sunset and nightfall. In Muslim countries these times are set aside as official breaks.
2. Usury (charging interest on loans) and games of chance are forbidden.
3. Muslims must give Alms to the poor.
4. They must observe a strict fast during the month of Ramadan. They are not allowed to eat or drink between sunrise and sunset.
5. They should attempt a Pilgrimage to the 'Ka'aba in Mecca' known as the Haj.

Food

Muslims are strictly forbidden to drink alcohol. Eating of pork is totally prohibited, so porcine insulin is unacceptable to Muslims; human insulin should be considered instead. Muslims eat only halal meat – any meat not from an animal killed by draining its blood while alive is prohibited.

Festivals

The Muslim year is divided into 12 lunar months, alternating between 29 and 30 days. Every festival is approximately 10 days earlier than the previous year.

- *Moharram:* an anniversary of the killing of the prophet's grandson Hussein. It is celebrated by Shi'I Muslims.
- *Ramadan:* birthday of the prophet Mohammed. A strict fast is practised from the first day until day 21 which is called the night of prayer.
- *Eid-ul-Fitr:* 2½-day festival to mark the end of Ramadan.
- *Eid-ul-Azho:* 3-day celebration of completion of pilgrimage to Mecca.
- *Mawild Al-Nabi:* the birthday of the prophet Mohammed (mostly in June).
- *Layat Al-Qadr (night):* day 26 of Ramadan.

Sikhism

The word Sikh is derived from the Sanskrit word for 'disciple'. The Sikhs are a most recognisable community all over the world: beards and turbans give Sikhs a very distinctive appearance. They represent about 2% of the population of India.

Sikhism emerged in the fifteenth century as a reformed sect to Hinduism, offering a common philosophy of humanism to Hindus and Muslims by the Guru Nanak. It developed further to self-identity and religion.

Beliefs

Sikhs believe in the openness of God, rejecting idolatry and worship of objects or images. Guru Nanak opposed discrimination on the grounds of caste, and believed 'God is One', formless, eternal and beyond description; God is present everywhere (Omnipresent) and visible to everyone.

The belief in the Hindu concept of Maya (wealth) was transformed into an unreal value commonly held by the world. Salvation depended on accepting the nature of God and true harmony of Divine order. They have the following requirements:

- Belief: worship, meditating by repeating God's name (*Nam*)
- Giving charity (*Dan*)
- Bathing (*Ishnan*)
- *Gurudhwara:* temple, a gateway to Guru
- *Gurugranth:* a religious scripture. Most families will have a *Gurugranth* and a shrine at home.

Every Sikh man has five 'Ks':

1. *Kesh* (uncut hair)
2. *Kangha* (comb)
3. *Kirpan* (dagger or a small sword)
4. *Kara* (steel bangle)
5. *Kacha* (boxer shorts).

Food

The temple, *Gurudhwara,* serves three free vegetarian meals with chapattis (*Langer*) every day all year round. These contain high fibre and starch. Desserts are invariably made of full cream milk, dry nuts and sugar. Sikhs do not eat beef.

Karah (*Prasad*) is an offering to Guru and served to people visiting the temple. It is made with ghee (melted butter), dry nuts and full cream milk. It is worth asking an Asian patient with diabetes how much is consumed.

Festivals

- *Baisakhi-Sikhs:* New Year celebrated with prayers and exchange of presents.
- *Guru Nanak:* festival.
- *Diwali:* celebrated by prayer, exchange of presents and distribution of sweets to friends and relatives.

All these festivals are associated with enjoyment and overindulgence in highly saturated carbohydrate sweets, syrups, dairy products and fried foods.

Judaism

It must also be remembered that people of the Jewish faith have dietary and other requirements. If a presenting patient is Jewish (and particularly of the orthodox faith) then it must be borne in mind that they will eat kosher food. There are many different levels of orthodoxy among the Jews, including:

- Mainstream orthodox
- Ultra orthodox (belonging to sects such as the Lubavitch)
- Reform
- Liberal.

The different levels differ in their adherence to the various rules and regulations set down by Judaism, concerning all sorts of things from eating kosher food, keeping a kosher home (separate sinks for milk and meat), to not working, travelling or carrying money on the Sabbath or festivals.

Beliefs

Judaism is the founding monotheistic religion, with one god (Yahweh or Elohim). Orthodox Jews pray three times a day – in the morning, early afternoon and evening – and prayers are said before every meal, and more or less before many activities. The bible (Torah) is taken literally by Orthodox Jews but there are many interpretative texts (e.g. the Mishnah) which are used to deal with secular issues. Orthodox Jewish men wear fringed garments under their clothes and keep their heads covered at all times. Orthodox Jewish women must wear long-sleeved dresses or blouses and skirts/dresses to their mid-calf; married women wear wigs and often keep their heads covered. Like Muslims, Jews are expected to give money or alms to charity.

Food

Kosher meat (like halal meat in Islam) is from an animal that has been killed in such a way that the blood drains from the body; a rabbi is present at the time of killing to give the seal of kashrut. Orthodox Jews do not eat pork, meat from animals with cloven hooves and shellfish. They also must not eat meat and dairy products together, or even use the same cutlery and crockery for the two products. Ultra orthodox families will have two sinks, two fridges and even two ovens in their kitchens. Many will also not eat anything that has been prepared in any place that does not adhere to kashrut. Note that use of 'animal' or 'natural' insulin could be prohibited under such rules, although Judaism always has waivers for avoiding anything that could be life threatening.

Festivals

- *Rosh Hashannah*: the Jewish new year – celebrated with such delicacies as honey cake.
- *Yom Kippur*: this is the Day of Atonement and involves fasting (including no drink or even toothbrushing) from sunset to an hour after sunset on the next day. Children under 13 and pregnant women (and anyone with health problems) are exempt.
- *Sukkot*: harvest festival – celebrated with lots of fruit and vegetables and the orthodox Jews eat their meals in a roofless booth built outdoors.
- *Simchat Torah*: the giving of the law.
- *Chanucah*: an 8-day celebration of the fight against the Greeks in the last

century BC, when a small jar of oil kept the everlasting light burning for 8 days. Traditional to eat foods cooked in oil: doughnuts, potato pancakes.

- *Purim*: festival of Esther; poppy seed cakes are traditionally eaten.
- *Passover*: celebration of the exodus from Egypt under Moses; lasts 8 days and no leavened food must be eaten for the duration (matzos are the unleavened bread consumed).
- *Shavuot*: festival of weeks (Pentecost is based on this festival). Traditional to eat diary products.
- There are many other minor fast days and festivals which are usually kept only by Orthodox Jews; as with the Sabbath all festivals start (and finish) at sunset.

The widespread availability and use of human insulin in the developed world means that there is now no problem for Jews (as well as people of other religious faiths) in accepting treatment with insulin (whether type 1 or type 2 treated with insulin). This may not be the case in developing countries, where insulin:

- may not be available at all
- supplies are limited
- species and type are not guaranteed
- strength is other than 100 U/ml
- may not be prescribed for cultural reasons.

African–Caribbean

African–Caribbean people are the second largest ethnic minority group in the UK. They have a high prevalence of diabetes (three to four times higher than in the white population), and poor outcomes from the disease. There is a notable difference in the outcome of diabetes in the African–Caribbean community, with a higher incidence of stroke and of end-stage renal failure than in the diabetic community as whole.

As there has not been much research on the group's health beliefs and experiences, there is a lack of specifically focused patient material. Health care professionals should try to address the health practices and beliefs of this group, so that they can make informed decisions on how they manage their condition.

Beliefs

The cultural understandings of Caribbean people are important because they can be used to interpret signs of illness and guide the selection of treatments, as well as evaluate the efficacy of these treatments.

There can be vast differences in how biomedicine and Caribbean people understand the functioning of the human body. Caribbean people have distinct beliefs about blood – this can lead to fasting and taking laxatives.

Caribbean people often categorise blood as 'good' or 'bad' – and this categorisation is more likely among older people and people with diabetes.

Most describe 'bad blood' as blood from a sick person – it is viewed as an index of poor health, often as a result of not eating properly.

Suggested ways of keeping blood 'good' include healthy eating, exercising, taking laxatives and home remedies such as vinegar, onions, garlic and cod liver oil. Many of these are positive practices, which can be incorporated into a diabetes management plan.

There may also be a reluctance, especially among elder members of the community, to have blood tests, because these can be seen as 'harmful'.

Food

Health care professionals have often reported their perception that obesity is viewed in positive terms within the African–Caribbean community. However, recent research shows that this does not appear to be the case – having a normal BMI is associated with health and attractiveness.

There does seem to be, however, a great unawareness of the link between obesity and the onset of diabetes. Only 4% of interviewees in a recent study mentioned a possible link between diabetes and obesity – all of whom had diabetes themselves.

It is important to make your African–Caribbean patients aware of this link, and to encourage them to eat healthily.

12

Hot and cold foods

In many communities around the world it is believed that certain foods are 'hot' whereas others are 'cold'. The hot or cold nature of foods bears no relation to the temperature or the spiciness of the dish. It is believed to be an inherent property of the food, supposedly giving rise to physical effects in the body.

Hot foods are supposed to raise the body temperature, excite the emotions and increase activity. Cold foods are believed to impart strength, cool the body and also to cause cheerfulness.

Normally a diet containing hot and cold foods would be consumed. However, during certain illnesses and in certain conditions, preference will be given to the nature of the foods.

Some of the foods with their hot and cold properties are listed in Table 12.1.

Table 12.1 Examples of the 'hot' and 'cold' foods

Food group	Hot	Cold
Cereals		Wheat, rice
Green leafy vegetables		All
Root vegetables	Carrot, onion	Potatoes
Other vegetables	Capsicum, pepper, aubergine or bringle	Cucumber, beans, cauliflower, marrow, gourd, ladies fingers (okra), etc.
Fruits	Dates, mango, pawpaw or papaya	All other fruits, e.g. apples, oranges, melons, etc.
Animal products	Meats, chicken, mutton, fish, eggs	
Milk products		Milk and cream, curds or yoghurt, buttermilk
Pulses	Lentils	Bangalgram or chickpea, greengram, peas, redgram
Nuts		All types, including ground or peanuts, cashew nuts
Spices and condiments	Chillies, green and red powder, cinnamon, clove, garlic, ginger, mustard, nutmeg pepper	Coriander, cumin, cardamom, fennel, tamarind
Oils	Mustard	Butter, coconut oil, ground nut oil
Miscellaneous	Tea, coffee, honey, jaggery or brown sugar	

Checklist for African–Asian patients with diabetes
- They are different people from different lands
- They have different cultures and customs; recognise their social and family needs
- English is not their first language – be patient, give them time and listen
- They have different customs: betel chewing, smoking and alcohol
- They have different religions; understanding and respect will be appreciated
- They have different etiquettes, and need extra sensitivity towards history taking/examination
- They have different dietary habits/beliefs: pork or beef is forbidden; the hierarchy in the household may also be significant
- They believe in 'hot' and 'cold' foods
- They use traditional/herbal medicines
- They can receive dietary advice from Diabetes UK
- Remind them to consult their doctor/nurse at the earliest signs of complications
- Doctors/nurses are available to help them and are sensitive to their needs

Food modification and dietary advice

Diabetes UK recommendations accommodate the dietary culture and preferences of the African–Asian population. The general rules apply and should be individually tailored to the person, religion, culture and family circumstances. Specific advice and recipes can be obtained from Diet and Information Services at Diabetes UK.

Many African–Asian people with diabetes constantly use various types of traditional/herbal medicines in conjunction with their therapeutic medications. These herbal medicines are mostly vegetables (Karela or guard – *memordicca carrantia* has a proven insulin-like substance). They are easily available in this country and most have potent hypoglycaemic properties. In fact also available in this country are some tablets and concentrated juices of these traditional medicines. Most of the tablets have four or five ingredients, some of which are hepatotoxic.

It is important to ask any African–Asian diabetic patient whether he or she is taking any of the above medications.

Further reading

Brent Health Education (1986). *Religion and Culture: A Guide to Religious and Culture Beliefs.*

Govindji A (1991). Dietary advice for the Asian Diabetic. *Practical Diabetes* **8**(5): 202–3.

Patroe L (2001). *An Executive Summary of the Diabetes Development Fund for Black and Minority Ethnic Communities in the North West of England.* London: Diabetes UK.

Scott P (2001). Caribbean people's health beliefs about the body and their implications for diabetes management: a South London Study. *Practical Diabetes International* **18** (3): 94–8.

13 Education for self-management

- Reasons for 'learning', 'understanding' and 'doing' gaps
- Assessment for diabetes self-management and education
- Getting the message across
- Complementary therapies

Diabetes education encompasses all aspects of clinical care and is integral to it, for the person with diabetes, for those close to him or her, and for all health care providers involved. The Diabetes Education Consultation Section of the International Diabetes Federation has published *International Consensus Standards of Practice for Diabetes Education* (1997), providing key elements and a framework by which structure, process and outcome standards for diabetes education can be measured at basic and optimal levels.

Living with diabetes requires knowledge and experience, built up over time. The level and pace of learning vary greatly between individuals. It is important for health care professionals to appreciate the gaps between 'learning', 'understanding' and 'doing' and why such gaps occur.

Reasons for 'learning', 'understanding' and 'doing' gaps

The newly diagnosed person

Considerable shock often accompanies the newly diagnosed person with diabetes. A sense of bereavement is felt, caused by the loss of health and fear of the unknown or of the future. This sense of shock and fear may also be felt by relatives and have a considerable impact on a whole family. It is at this time that a great deal of information may be passed to the person concerned, much of which is unnecessary at this stage and may even be counterproductive and confusing.

Preconceived ideas

Experiences of diabetes previously learned from family members or friends may have been negative and even horrific, resulting in extreme fear and concern. This may block any constructive discussion regarding self-management at an early stage.

Fear of living with diabetes

Preconceived ideas may lead to particular concerns of living with diabetes, such as restrictions in eating, drinking and everyday activities. Worries may be expressed regarding employment, driving, travel, holidays and, in younger people, the implications of diabetes on attending college, leaving home, starting work and starting a family.

Culture

Culture and personal health beliefs have a considerable bearing on attitudes to disease and coping with a life-long progressive condition, such as diabetes. In certain societies, being overweight in a woman is regarded as beautiful and desirable, in others the opposite is true. The diagnosis of diabetes in some cultures may place the person concerned into a 'sick role', rendering the concept of living a healthy life with diabetes difficult to grasp. For further details of how to deal with cultural aspects, see Chapter 12 'Aspects of culture relating to diabetes care'.

Fear of long-term complications of diabetes

Again preconceived ideas and some previous knowledge of diabetes may result in extreme concern (even a morbid fear) of complications, particularly regarding eyes and blindness, feet and amputation.

Physical difficulties

Elderly people in particular may have problems with physical disability and suffer a reduction in their mobility. The sight, hearing and senses of touch, smell and taste may become less acute with age.

Mental difficulties

People with learning disabilities, mental illness or disability require particular care in their management. Much of the burden of their diabetes and concerns over its progression will fall to relatives or carers, who require special support.

The ageing process affects the memory as well as the ability to take in information and act on it. As people become older, they may appear to cope quite well with living with diabetes but be reluctant to change certain habits built up over a lifetime.

Literacy and education

Literacy is assumed, both in our own society and in others. An illiterate person should not be deemed stupid; in fact the reverse may be true. Compensation by the person for illiteracy may be such that the problem is effectively disguised.

Educational levels, particularly regarding how the body works, should not be taken for granted. A highly intelligent and well-educated person is often assumed to be knowledgeable and coping when, in fact, the diagnosis may be denied or fear of complications may lead to obsessional monitoring and control of blood glucose levels ruling the person's life.

Language

Language is obviously a barrier to communication where English is not the mother tongue. It is important that appropriate translation methods are used, such as help from family members if appropriate, health link workers or a telephone translation scheme such as Language Line (available in some health districts). Contact with local ethnic minority groups may also generate local interest in diabetes, translating expertise and materials into the appropriate language.

The greatest difficulty with language used by health care professionals is the use of medical terminology which is either not understood or misunderstood and, in most instances, is inappropriate. Most people are grateful for a simple non-technical explanation and will enquire further if this is insufficient.

Attitude

An attitude is described as a 'settled mode of thinking and behaviour'. In diabetes, this is governed by what happens at diagnosis and immediately thereafter. Good management at this stage will set the scene for the future attitude towards diabetes and self-care. Positive ongoing support, which is non-judgemental and responsive to concerns expressed by the person with diabetes, will help to reinforce the person's desire to look after him- or herself.

Information giving

There are six main problems of information giving as identified by people with diabetes. These are:

- *Incorrect information* – where facts given about diabetes are wrong. It is much better for the health care professional to admit ignorance and offer to find out the correct information.
- *Inconsistent information* – where several health care professionals are involved and different educational messages are received, giving a confusing picture.
- *Too much information* – where too many messages are given, often at the same time, particularly at or near the diagnosis.
- *Too little information* – where the information supplied or requested is insufficient for the person concerned to find it useful or helpful.
- *Inappropriate information* – where the information given is not appropriate to the diabetes requirements or the age and lifestyle of the person concerned.
- *Lack of up-to-date information* – where information is given at diagnosis or when specifically requested and no further or new information is offered. In order to avoid this, individual or group education programmes should be planned, recorded and new information offered as soon as it is learned by the doctor, nurse or other health care professional involved. One of the main reasons for this is the lack of continuing education by heath care professionals.

Motivational interviewing

Most people don't like being told what to do; their personal freedom is threatened. As health care professionals we need to avoid the message that 'I am the expert and I'm going to tell you how to run your life'. It is not enough to know what people with diabetes should change in their life in order to keep their diabetes 'under control'. We also need to know how we can help our patients make the changes that they want to make. One process that can help is called 'motivational interviewing'.

> Motivational interviewing is a particular way to help people recognize and do something about their present or potential problems. It is particularly useful with people who are reluctant to change and ambivalent about changing. It is intended to help resolve ambivalence and to get a person moving along the path to change. For some people, this is all they really need. Once they are unstuck, no longer immobilized by conflicting motivations, they have all the skills and resources they need in order to make lasting change. All they need is a relatively brief motivational boost.
>
> Miller and Rollnick (1991)

Home, work and social life

Home, work and social life influence the control and even the progression of diabetes. Unemployment, financial concerns and loneliness may be hidden, but may be the reason for a change in eating habits, shoes of a poorer quality, disinterest or depression.

Opportunities in careers, employment, in sport and other common life experiences may be over-shadowed by the stigma of diabetes.

Lifestyle changes

Leaving home for the first time, a change of home or job, retirement or the loss of a partner may cause a major change in attitude and behaviour. Extra support and further education may be needed at these times.

Assessment for diabetes self-management and education

This should take place at annual review and if appropriate at every routine review. The assessment (by enquiry) should include:

- Demographic information/changes
- Family status/changes
- Employment status/changes
- Medical history/changes
- Lifestyle history/changes
- Diabetes management/changes.

In addition, at diagnosis (or for a person with diabetes who has recently joined the practice), the assessment (by enquiry or observation) should include the following:

- Family history of diabetes
- Preconceived ideas of diabetes
- Knowledge of diabetes/complications
- Circumstances surrounding diagnosis
- Feelings surrounding diagnosis (patient)
- Feelings surrounding diagnosis (family/carers)
- Culture/language
- Physical difficulties
- Mental difficulties

- Literacy/education
- Attitude to diabetes.

Getting the message across

Initially, education about diabetes in the general practice situation is best provided individually after assessment, although it can be helpful for a newly diagnosed person to meet someone who has had the condition for a time and has come to terms with it. In association with information provided, the practice should be able to offer the following resources (see resources list, Appendix VIII):

- Titles of books/a book loan scheme
- Booklets, leaflets (available from pharmaceutical companies or Diabetes UK)
- Address/telephone number – Diabetes UK
- Address/telephone number – local branch, Diabetes UK
- Local information regarding diabetes care and associated services (dietetic/chiropody [podiatry])
- Supportive agencies
- Social services.

Whenever possible, education provided should be backed up with written information or the help to obtain it.

Once the service for people with diabetes is established in the practice, group education sessions may prove valuable, the people with diabetes bringing along a relative or friend.

Group sessions for eight to ten people (more than this may be too inhibiting) can be held around a cup of tea or appropriate snack lunch (financed by sponsorship from an appropriate pharmaceutical company, if practice policy supports this).

Information technology and health education

Individual and group health education programmes can now be enhanced by creative information technology (IT) packages using multimedia techniques. *Learning Diabetes (insulin treated)* and *Learning Diabetes (non-insulin treated)* are a new approach to diabetes education developed by Dr John Day and Dr Gerry Rayman of the Ipswich Diabetes Centre and their colleagues, in collaboration with multimedia experts and many people with diabetes and their families. They are multimedia patient education programmes produced as a package called 'Managing Your Health' by Interactive Eurohealth (see Appendix

VIII). These programmes and other such multimedia approaches allow interaction, problem-solving and a way of learning that is acceptable and user-friendly to people of all ages. They may also be a focus for discussion in education programmes for people with diabetes and their families, in addition to their use in the education of health care providers, individually or in groups.

As the general population logs into the internet, people with diabetes and those caring for them can join supportive diabetes networks across the world as well as accessing the very latest developments in diabetes research and technology.

It is important that IT is used sensitively and *not instead of* the personal touch. It is a tool for the development of understanding and should, whenever possible, be planned into a structured, monitored and evaluated diabetes education programme.

Group diabetes education in the practice

Organisation

- Selecting group to be invited (i.e. people treated with diet, tablets or insulin)
- Selecting members of the primary care team to be involved (and group facilitator)
- Deciding time, length and place of session
- Arranging tea/coffee/snacks
- Setting objectives for the session (to be agreed by participants)
- Inviting participants (with a minimum of 2 weeks' notice – Fig. 13.1)
- Designing a simple evaluation form for participants to complete following the session (Fig. 13.2).

13

Invitations can be given verbally to people attending the diabetes clinic if the group session is planned well ahead (to save telephone calls/stamps). Alternatively, a letter of invitation may be sent (Fig. 13.1).

Fig. 13.1 Sample letter of invitation for a group diabetes session

Practice Telephone No.: 222333
The Medical Practice
Woolley End Road
Airedale Edge
SHEFFIELD
South Yorkshire S2 3AB

January 2001

Mrs P Johnson
The Tannery
Black Terrace
SHEFFIELD S1 1XX

Dear Mrs Johnson

Re: Diabetes Care

We are planning to hold a lunchtime session for people with diabetes to discuss:

- Planning meals
- Testing for sugar
- Other topics, as required.

on Wednesday 18 April 2001, at 12.30pm.

The session will finish at 2 pm and a snack lunch will be provided.

You and your husband are warmly invited to attend. If you are unable to come, we would be grateful if you would let us know.

Yours sincerely

Dr A Smith (General Practitioner)   Mrs M Jones (Practice Nurse)

Fig. 13.2 Sample evaluation form for use following a group diabetes session

The Medical Practice
Woolley End Road
Airedale Edge
SHEFFIELD
South Yorkshire S2 3AB

Diabetes care – group session

Date:

In order to assess today's session, we would be grateful if you would fill in this form. Thank you.

Please delete the answer that does not apply to you and make your own comments.

1. Are you   A person with diabetes?

_____ A relative?

_____ A friend?

2. Did you receive sufficient notice to attend today's session?

YES/NO

3. Meal planning

(a) Was the topic covered sufficiently for you?

YES/NO

(b) Were there aspects of the topic not covered?

YES/NO

(c) What aspects of this topic would you have like discussed further? Please write them down:

_____
_____
_____
_____

Fig. 13.2 contd

4. Testing for sugar

(a) Was the topic covered enough for you?

YES/NO

(b) Were there aspects of the topic not covered?

YES/NO

(c) What aspects of this topic would you have liked to discuss further? Please write them down:

5. What other topics discussed did you find useful in the session? Please write them down:

_____
_____
_____
_____

6. Did you find that today's session helped you to understand more about living with diabetes?

YES/NO

7. Would you be interested in attending further group sessions relating to diabetes care?

YES/NO

8. Do you have any suggestions for future sessions? Please write them down:

_____
_____
_____
_____

Thank you for filling in this form.

Facilitating the session

This includes:

- Preparation of room
- Greeting participants
- Domestic arrangements (coats/toilets, etc.)
- Introductions
- Arrangements for tea/coffee/snacks
- Stating the aims of the session and discussing these with participants
- Identifying topics requested by participants
- Introducing topics
- Allowing discussion to progress around topics
- Time-keeping
- Summarising session
- Organising evaluation form to be completed
- Arranging follow-up/further session
- Dealing with any personal problems identified during the session
- Supervising departure of participants
- Clearing up
- Discussing evaluation forms and session with other members of the team
- Recording education session in practice and patient records.

'Getting the message across' in diabetes education, whether to individuals or to groups, involves the following:

- Discussing and planning education concerned with the person with diabetes/relative/carer
- Listening
- Hearing what is being said
- 'Picking up' hidden worries and difficulties
- Responding to questions
- Dealing with urgent problems
- Asking the right questions in the right way
- Being non-judgemental
- 'Staging' information
- Providing small pieces of information at one time
- Obtaining feedback on information given
- Summarising information given
- Demonstrating practical skills
- Observing practical skills learned
- Being positive, encouraging and supportive
- Recording information given and skills learned

13

- Discussing and planning further education with the person with diabetes/relative/carer.

Complementary therapies

People with diabetes and their relatives/carers may have had experiences of, or heard about, help through complementary therapies. As long as all involved understand that it is essential for people with diabetes to continue with their treatment, such complementary therapies may benefit people with diabetes. The therapies available are extensive and the box gives addresses of organisations that could be contacted for further information. It is advisable for people with diabetes to discuss the situation with those involved in their care before starting any such therapy.

Aromatherapy Organisations Council
PO Box 19834, London SE25 6WF
Tel: 020 8251 7912
Fax: 020 8251 7942
Website: www.aromatherapy-uk.org

Association of Qualified Curative Hypnotherapists
10 Balaclava Road, King's Heath, Birmingham B14 7SG
Tel: 0121 441 1775
Website: www.aqch.org

British Acupuncture Council
63 Jeddo Road, London W12 9HQ
Tel: 020 8735 0400
Fax: 020 8735 0404
Website: www.acupuncture.org.uk

British Herbal Medicine Association
Sun House, Church Street, Stroud, Glos GL5 1JS
Tel: 01453 751389
Fax: 01453 751402

British Homeopathic Association
15 Clerkenwell Close, London EC1R 0AA
Tel: 020 7566 7800
Fax: 020 7566 7815
Website: www.trusthomeopathy.org

British Medical Acupuncture Society
12 Marbury House, Higher Whitley, Warrington, Cheshire WA4 4QW
Tel: 01925 730727
Fax: 01925 730492
Website: www.medical-acupuncture.co.uk

British Society of Medical and Dental Hypnosis
National Office, 17 Keppel View Road, Kimberworth, Rotherham S61 2AR
Tel: 01709 554558
Fax: 01709 554558

British Wheel of Yoga
25 Jermyn Street, Sleaford, Lincs NG34 7RU
Tel: 01529 306851
Fax: 01529 303233
Website: www.bwy.org.uk

Council for Complementary and Alternative Medicine
63 Jeddo Road, London W12 9HQ
Tel: 020 8735 0632

13

Institute for Complementary Medicine
PO Box 194, London SE16 7QZ
Tel: 020 7237 5165
Fax: 020 7237 5175
Website: www.icmedicine.co.uk

International Federation of Aromatherapists
182 Chiswick High Road, London W4 1PP
Tel: 020 8742 2605
Fax: 020 8742 2606
Website: www.int-fed-aromatherapy.co.uk

National Institute of Medical Herbalists
56 Longbrook Street, Exeter, Devon EX4 6AH
Tel: 01392 426022
Fax: 01392 498963
Website: www.NIMH.org.uk

Relaxation for Living
12 New Street, Chipping Norton, Oxon OX7 5LF
Tel: 01983 868166

Society of Homeopaths
4a Artizan Road
Northampton NN1 4HU
Tel: 01604 621400
Fax: 01604 622622
Website: www.homeopathy-soh.org

Yoga for Health Foundation
Ickwell Bury, Biggleswade, Beds SG18 9EF
Tel: 01767 627271
Fax: 01767 627266
Website: yogaforhealthfoundation.co.uk

Further reading

IDF Consultative Section on Diabetes Education (1997). *International Consensus Standards of Practice for Diabetes Education.* London: Class Publishing.

Miller WR, Rollnick S (1991). *Motivational Interviewing. Preparing People to change Addictive Behavior.* New York: Guilford Press.

Walker R (1998). Diabetes reflecting on empowerment. *Nursing Standard* **12**(23): 49–56.

14

Living with diabetes: information requirements

■ After confirmation of diagnosis
■ Living with diabetes (further information)

These are 'key' points only, providing a focus for discussion. The information should be 'staged' to the appropriate time, or provided when questions are asked. Information given must be recorded (for legal reasons).

After confirmation of diagnosis

Understanding diabetes

■ Preconceived ideas/fear of complications
■ Causes
■ Symptoms
■ Treatment/effect of treatment/benefits
■ Preconceived ideas – living with diabetes.

Dietary advice

■ 'Diabetic foods' to be avoided
■ Assessment of food/meals (family)
■ Targets for weight control (personal)
■ Dietary changes required/discussed
■ Meal planning (family)
■ Contact/referral – dietitian.

Care provision (where, how and who?)

■ In general practice
■ In hospital diabetes clinic

- Shared by general practice and hospital diabetes clinic
- Care provided in specialist clinics (eyes/feet)
- Changes in care provision
- Importance of regular review
- Importance of annual review.

Contact numbers

- Telephone number of general practice/hospital diabetes services
- Use of contact numbers, if problems
- Use of contact numbers, if unwell.

Living with diabetes (further information – as appropriate)

Medication (oral hypoglycaemic agents)

- Name of drug
- Reason for use of drug
- Effect of drug
- Side effects of drug
- Dose of drug
- When to take drug
- Hypoglycaemic risk of drug (if a sulphonylurea)
- Symptoms of hypoglycaemia
- Prevention of hypoglycaemia
- Treatment of hypoglycaemia
- Continuation of drug supplies – ordering of prescription – notice required by practice
- Prescription exemption – FP92A – signed by doctor.

Insulin

- Name, species, type, dose, effect of insulin
- Giving the injection (how, where and when?)
- Spare insulin (in fridge)
- Care and disposal of syringes, needles, pens
- Risk of hypoglycaemia
- Symptoms of hypoglycaemia
- Prevention of hypoglycaemia (carriage of glucose, identification)

- Treatment of hypoglycaemia (Hypostop/glucagon)
- Contact number to ring – if problems; diabetes nurse specialist/clinic/centre
- Insulin dose adjustments (when and how)
- Continuation of insulin and supplies – ordering of prescription – notice required by practice
- Prescription exemption – FP92A – signed by doctor.

Hyperglycaemia

- Symptoms
- Prevention
- Action to take.

Other medication taken (e.g. steroids)

- Effect on diabetes control
- Action to take if control affected (e.g. seek advice from doctor).

Illness rules

- Continue with medication/insulin, increasing dose as advised by primary care team
- Drink plenty of liquid (tea, water)
- Test urine/blood 2–4 hourly
- If vomiting or illness persists **contact doctor.**

Urine testing

- Reasons for testing (benefits)
- Demonstration of test strips
- How to test
- When to test and how often
- The meaning of the test in relation to blood glucose levels (of the individual)
- The renal threshold
- Recording tests
- Action to take if urine glucose levels high
- Prescription for strips (unless treated with diet alone).

Blood glucose monitoring

- Reasons for testing (benefits)
- Demonstration of test strips

14

- Demonstration of equipment for testing
- How to test
- When to test
- Interpretation of test results
- Recording tests
- Action to take if blood glucose levels outside negotiated target range
- Prescription for strips.

Alcohol

- Risk of hypoglycaemia (with insulin and sulphonylureas)
- Drinking guidelines (Diabetes UK recommendations)
- Dangers when driving (especially with added risk of hypoglycaemia)
- Risk of weight gain (and hyperglycaemia).

Smoking

- General risks of smoking
- Added risk of smoking and diabetes
- Encouragement/support to stop smoking
- Follow-up support if smoking stopped.

Blood pressure

- What blood pressure means
- Importance of annual blood pressure check
- Importance of blood pressure control in association with diabetes
- Value of weight reduction, salt restriction and increased exercise, if blood pressure raised
- Alcohol restriction and caffeine reduction may also be helpful before drug treatment is used
- If drugs for raised blood pressure are prescribed, it is important that they are taken regularly
- Effect of hypertensive drugs.

Special occasions, celebrations, eating out

- Important that these are enjoyed
- Important to know to adjust insulin – for enjoyment!
- Blood glucose levels will be higher if more food or sweet foods are taken
- Urine tests/blood tests may demonstrate higher blood glucose levels
- Urine/blood glucose levels should settle in a day or two
- Alcohol may lower blood glucose levels.

Annual review

Importance and reasons for annual review – opportunity for:

- Overview of general health/lifestyle
- Overview of diabetes and education
- Review of targets for weight, blood pressure and blood glucose levels (explain HbA1c)
- Review of laboratory results
- Medical examination
- Sight test
- Screening for diabetic retinopathy
- Examination of feet and shoes
- Urine checked for presence of protein.

Eye care and screening

- Sight test
- Check annual visit to optician for free eye test. Importance of correct spectacles
- Pupils will be dilated before backs of eyes are examined by doctor
- Each eye checked by doctor using ophthalmoscope
- Report any eye problems immediately (to practice).

Foot and shoe care

- Examine feet and shoes regularly (use a mirror if necessary)
- Look for sore areas or cracks, especially between the toes
- Report problems immediately (to practice)
- Keep feet clean (regular washing and careful drying)
- Keep toe nails trimmed (a chiropodist/podiatrist may be needed)
- Avoid extremes of heat/cold
- Make sure new shoes fit (length, width and depth)
- Make sure socks, stockings or tights fit
- Avoid garters.

Chiropody/podiatry (may be required)

- For toe nails to be trimmed
- For treatment of corn, callus
- For insoles or special shoes
- For regular care.

Family planning advice

■ Fertility is not impaired in diabetes except in the presence of severe renal disease.

■ Oral contraception is effective (1% failure rate).

■ Oral contraceptives should not be used in women with diabetes in the following circumstances:
   ◆ older women
   ◆ overweight women
   ◆ those with small- or large-vessel disease
   ◆ those with a family history of vascular disease
   ◆ smokers.

■ High-dose combined oral contraceptives should not be used in women with a previous history of gestational diabetes or who have diabetes.

■ Low-dose combined oral contraceptives may be used in the short term (with monitoring of blood glucose levels and blood pressure).

■ Low-dose progestogens may be used (they may not be so well tolerated or effective).

■ Intrauterine contraceptive devices can be used except in women with a history of acute pelvic infection or pelvic inflammatory disease.

■ Barrier methods and sterilisation can be offered to all women with diabetes.

■ Vasectomy can be offered to men with diabetes.

Pre-conception

■ Blood glucose levels should be well controlled three months before conception

■ Pre-pregnancy counselling, education and support should be planned

■ Early referral is necessary.

Pregnancy

■ Continuing support and surveillance by obstetric and diabetes teams are necessary throughout pregnancy and in the postnatal period

■ Early referral is recommended

■ Dietary adjustments may be required during the establishment of breast feeding

■ Protection should be provided against rubella during pregnancy.

Hormone replacement therapy (HRT)

- HRT can and should be used in women with diabetes (oestrogens have a cardioprotective effect)
- Progestogens have an anti-insulin effect
- Blood glucose levels should be carefully monitored
- Insulin doses may need adjustment.

Erectile dysfunction

- Often a 'hidden problem' – embarrassing for the person with diabetes and the health care professional.
- Sensitive questioning and discussion should be instigated by educated health care professionals, whether the patient is seen by the primary care or the specialist team.
- Common in men with a long history of diabetes.
- May be the cause of marital difficulties.
- Failure to gain an erection may be caused by:
  - autonomic neuropathy
  - vascular dysfunction
  - psychological factors.
- Careful assessment for the underlying cause(s) is essential.
- Referral to a specialist diabetes/genitourinary team may be necessary.
- Treatment options:
  - counselling for both partners (may also be needed in conjunction with other treatment options)
  - vacuum therapy
  - intracavernosal injection therapy
  - transurethral alprostadil (MUSE)
  - sildenafil (Viagra) – can be prescribed on the NHS for men with diabetes as well as for those with multiple sclerosis, spinal cord injury, prostate cancer, those undergoing treatment for renal failure and following radical pelvic surgery, severe pelvic injury and prostatectomy. Also for those with poliomyelitis, spinal bifida and Parkinson's disease. (Cardiovascular risk assessment and contraindications with other medication, e.g. nitrate therapy, should be observed before sildenafil is prescribed.)

Cervical screening

- Should be offered to women with diabetes.

14

Breast screening

■ Should be offered to women with diabetes.

Tetanus immunisation

■ Should be offered to people with diabetes.

Pneumococcal immunisation

■ Should be offered to anyone aged over two years in whom pneumococcal infection is likely to be more common or dangerous, and this includes people with diabetes mellitus, as well as those with chronic kidney, heart or lung disease.
■ It can be given together with influenza vaccine, although the pneumococcal vaccine is given as a single dose.

Influenza immunisation

■ Influenza may upset diabetes control (particularly in frail and elderly people)
■ Protection should be offered if not medically contraindicated
■ Diabetes control may be upset after flu immunisation
■ Extra monitoring is advisable
■ Medication or insulin therapy may require temporary adjustment.

Children and young people with diabetes

■ Require special care and management.
■ Parents need support.
■ Should be referred appropriately on diagnosis.
■ May have particular problems at certain stages of childhood and development (e.g. change of school, onset of puberty), requiring extra support.
■ Diabetes control can deteriorate quickly (especially during an illness). Urgent admission to hospital may be required.
■ All immunisations should be offered to children/young people with diabetes.
■ As adult life approaches, support and counselling are required in association with higher education, employment, social pressures, driving and living away from home for the first time.

Employment

- Safety of the person with diabetes and safety of other people (in association with hypoglycaemia) must be considered.
- People with diabetes (insulin treated) are not usually accepted for:
  - the armed forces
  - the police service
  - the merchant navy
  - the fire brigade
  - the prison service
  - working at heights
  - deep sea diving
  - working on oil rigs
  - coal face working
  - truck or bus driving.
- People with diabetes may not be recruited as pilots, on the flight deck or in air traffic control.
- Shift work can be accommodated with flexible insulin regimens.
- Those treated with diet alone, or diet and medication, can undertake most occupations (as the risk of hypoglycaemia is small), although some blanket bans on recruitment still apply.

Sport and leisure

- Safety of the person with diabetes and safety of others (in association with hypoglycaemia) must be considered.
- Risk factors should always be taken into account by those treated with insulin.
- An accompanying person is a sensible precaution.
- A few sports apply restrictions to people with diabetes.
- Extra food and/or an insulin dose reduction may be needed relating to degree of activity.
- Extra food (if treated with medication) may be needed relating to degree of activity.
- Possibility of delayed hypoglycaemia (after strenuous activity). This may occur many hours later.
- Symptoms, prevention and treatment of hypoglycaemia in association with sport and leisure activities.

14

Driving

Car driving licences

■ Car driving licences can be held by people with diabetes.

■ The DVLA in Swansea must be informed of the presence of diabetes and any treatment change (e.g. from diet alone to medication or medication to insulin), except if the diabetes is diet controlled. This is required by law. *Note:* this information must be provided and recorded. The decision to follow this advice is the responsibility of the individual concerned.

■ Licences are renewed every one, two or three years depending on health (of people treated with insulin).

■ Licence renewal forms are sent automatically before the expiry date. There is no fee for renewal.

■ Licence renewal is granted after completion of the form (including signed consent for the individual's doctor to be consulted by the DVLA, if required) by the person with diabetes.

■ A medical check may be requested by the DVLA.

■ Those treated with diet alone or tablets are not subject to licence restrictions (for diabetes). They can retain their 'until aged 70' privilege, but must inform the DVLA if there is any change to treatment.

■ The driver must inform his or her driving insurance company of the presence of diabetes.

■ Some insurance companies load the driver's premium. This should be challenged. It is sensible to 'shop around' because the Disability Discrimination Act 1995 has improved this situation. Diabetes UK Insurance Services can also offer motor insurance cover (see Appendix VIII).

Vocational driving licences

■ Vocational driving licences are required for Large Goods Vehicles (LGV) and Passenger Carrying Vehicles (PCV).

■ People with diabetes, whose condition is treated with diet alone, or diet and medication, and who are well controlled may hold these licences.

■ People with diabetes treated with diet and insulin may not hold these licences (even if they held a licence before starting insulin treatment). An exception to this rule is made only for those who have previously held a vocational licence issued by a licensing authority in the knowledge of their insulin treatment before 1991.

■ Holders of vocational driving licences must inform the DVLA on commencement of insulin treatment. *Note:* this information must be provided and recorded.

The decision to follow this advice is the responsibility of the individual concerned:

- If not followed, the licence will be revoked.
- There is, however, a statutory right of appeal (details are sent from the DVLA when the licence is revoked).
- General advice regarding appeals against the withdrawal of car and vocational driving licences can be obtained from Diabetes UK.
- People with visual impairment should not drive.
- People who have lost their warning signs of hypoglycaemia should not drive.
- Drivers should know the symptoms, prevention and treatment of hypoglycaemia.
- Sweets/biscuits should always be available in the vehicle.
- If hypoglycaemic warning signs occur, the driver should:
  - move as safely as possible to the side of the road
  - stop the car and remove the keys from the ignition
  - move to the passenger seat and take sweets/biscuits
  - resume driving **only** when safe to do so
  - have a substantial starchy snack or meal as soon as possible.

Life insurance policies

- As with motor insurance, life insurance is calculated according to age and state of health.
- A life assurance policy already held should not be affected by the diagnosis of diabetes. It is not necessary to declare the diabetes.
- If a new policy is taken out, the diabetes must be declared and the policy may be loaded. This can be challenged.
- Advice about sympathetic insurance companies can be obtained from Diabetes UK.

Travel and holidays

- Immunisation may be required. Exact details will depend on the country to be visited (available in the practice).
- Diabetes control may be temporarily affected (by immunisation).
- Travel insurance should include:
  - declaring diabetes (to obtain adequate cover)
  - checking extent of coverage
  - looking for a premium with a minimum coverage of £250,000
  - contacting Diabetes UK for further information if required.
- Obtain Form T1 (from local DSS office) – *The Travellers' Guide to Health.*
- Obtain Form E111 (from local DSS office) for medical care in EC countries.

- The following should be considered before travel:
  - ◆ identification (card/bracelet)
  - ◆ if travelling abroad, a doctor's letter may be helpful when carrying syringes/insulin (particularly at customs points)
  - ◆ travel sickness prevention
  - ◆ anti-diarrhoea medication
  - ◆ anti-malarial medication (if appropriate)
  - ◆ a supply of antibiotics
  - ◆ simple dressings
  - ◆ sufficient medication/insulin (insulin stored in a cool bag) and carried in hand luggage (U100 insulin is not available everywhere)
  - ◆ sufficient supplies of syringes/needle clipper (carried in hand luggage)
  - ◆ monitoring equipment (carried in hand luggage)
  - ◆ sunburn protection cream
  - ◆ sun hat
  - ◆ water purification tablets (if appropriate)
  - ◆ appropriate footwear
  - ◆ carriage of sweets/biscuits when travelling
  - ◆ contact Diabetes UK for details about specific countries/appropriateness of specific vaccines with insulin or oral hypoglycaemics.
- The following may also be helpful:
  - ◆ British Airways Travel Clinics Location Line
    (Recorded information line)
    Tel: 01276 685040
  - ◆ British Airways Travel Clinic
    Tel: 020 7637 9899
    Master Travellers' health Line
    (Recorded information line)
    0906 822 4100
    Travel advice line 0891 172111 (currently charged at 60p/minute) or 0906 708 8807 (charged at 50p/minute).
  - ◆ Liverpool School of Tropical Medicine
    Pembroke Place
    Liverpool L3 SQA
    Tel: 0151 708 9393

Dental care

- Regular dental checks are important
- Dental infections may disturb diabetes control
- A painful mouth may prevent eating (particularly poorly fitting dentures) and a subsequent risk of hypoglycaemia
- There is no financial help for people with diabetes, relating to dental care.

Further reading

Day J (1998). *Living with Diabetes: The BDA guide for those treated with insulin*. Chichester: John Wiley & Sons.

Day J (1998). *Living with Diabetes: The BDA guide for those treated with diet and exercise*. Chichester: John Wiley & Sons.

Foster M, Cole M (1996). *Impotence*. London: Martin Dunitz Ltd.

Price DE (2001). The management of erectile dysfunction in diabetes. *International Diabetes Monitor* 13(2): 6–9.

14

15 Monitoring and audit of practice diabetes care

- Clinical audit and evaluation
- Recommended minimum dataset for management of diabetes in primary care
- Chronic disease management – diabetes programme

Diabetes UK recommends these audit guidelines for diabetes management in primary care.

Clinical audit and evaluation

Clinical audit of practice-based diabetes services should be performed regularly. The primary health care team should select which criteria they wish to audit and agree the standards of care against which to audit the quality of care provided. Medical Audit Advisory Groups (MAAGs) can also play an important role in facilitating clinical audit in primary care. Many practices have Practice Audit Coordinators financed by MAAGs.

The accumulation of data at district, regional or national level, as recommended in the St Vincent Declaration, can enable the evaluation of the effectiveness of diabetes services in improving the health of people with diabetes.

The St Vincent Declaration specifies outcomes for which targets are set. Incidence rates for these outcomes are such that they can only usefully be interpreted at district, regional and national levels.

If data collected at practice level are to be aggregated, it is important to ensure standardisation of the data collected. A suggested minimum dataset for use in primary care is set out later in this chapter. There are many software systems for primary diabetes care now available. Primary care diabetes read codes have been introduced in 1997. Patients must be notified (under the Data Protection Act):

- That they are on a register (if the register is held outside the practice)
- About the purpose of the register and who has access to it
- That they have the right to refuse.

This process may be facilitated by the sending of information by practices to a district diabetes register for computer entry and analysis. Alternatively, if data are entered on practice computers, it should be in a format that can be analysed and amalgamated at district level.

As the outcomes for which targets are set in the St Vincent Declaration have long time scales, it is important to monitor measures of process, acute and intermediate outcomes and cardiovascular risk factors, and other markers of late complications so that progress in the shorter term can also be monitored.

Process measures

■ The level of ascertainment of patients with diagnosed diabetes.
■ The apparent prevalence of diabetes in the practice population can be compared with the expected prevalence, taking into account the age and ethnic make-up of the practice population. A low figure may suggest under-ascertainment.
■ The proportion of identified patients reviewed within the last year.
■ The proportion of identified patients in whom the following have been assessed within the last year:
  ◆ body mass index (BMI)
  ◆ dietary intake – by State-Registered Dietitian
  ◆ tobacco consumption
  ◆ urinalysis for proteinuria
  ◆ blood pressure
  ◆ glycated haemoglobin level (or fructosamine)
  ◆ serum lipids
  ◆ serum creatinine
  ◆ eyes: visual acuity and fundoscopy through dilated pupils
  ◆ feet: footwear, evidence of circulation problems and neuropathy.
■ The proportion of patients, identified as having the following problems, who are receiving appropriate management:
  ◆ smoking
  ◆ hypertension
  ◆ hyperlipidaemia
  ◆ eye problem
  ◆ renal problem
  ◆ foot problem.

Outcome measures

Acute outcomes

- Proportion requiring hospital admission for ketoacidosis within last year
- Proportion requiring professional attention for 'hypo' within last year
- Proportion of patients with cataract
- Proportion of patients with angina
- Proportion of patients with claudication
- Proportion of patients with symptomatic neuropathy
- Proportion of patients with impotence.

Pregnancy outcomes

- Abortion rates in women with diabetes: spontaneous miscarriages and terminations for congenital abnormality
- Stillbirth and perinatal mortality rates among infants of mothers with diabetes
- Incidence of congenital abnormalities.

Intermediate outcomes

- Pattern of glycaemic control for each treatment group.

Cardiovascular risk factors

- Proportion of patients who smoke
- Proportion of patients who take no exercise
- Proportion of patients with BMI > 30
- Proportion of patients with hypertension
- Proportion of patients with raised cholesterol
- Proportion of patients with raised triglycerides.

Markers of late complications

- Proportion of patients with proteinuria/microalbuminuria
- Proportion of patients with raised creatinine
- Proportion of patients with background and sight-threatening retinopathy
- Proportion of patients with absent foot pulses
- Proportion of patients with reduced vibration sense
- Proportion of patients with reduced pin-prick sensation
- Proportion of patients with foot ulceration.

15

Late outcomes

- Proportion of patients who have had a myocardial infarction
- Proportion of patients who have had a stroke
- Proportion of patients with visual impairment
- Proportion of patients with severe visual impairment
- Proportion of patients with end-stage renal failure
- Proportion of patients who have had an amputation: below/above ankle
- Age-specific mortality rates in people with diabetes.

Measures of health status, quality of life and patient satisfaction

- Psychological well-being
- Physical well-being
- Knowledge of diabetes
- Self-care performance
- Satisfaction with care
- Satisfaction with care delivery.

Questionnaire surveys are required to monitor these measures. Attendance rates at clinic and waiting times to be seen in clinic can be used as proxy measures for patient satisfaction.

Recommended minimum dataset for management of diabetes in primary care

Patient details

Name	NHS number	Date of birth	Sex

Address

Year of diagnosis	Ethnic origin

Annual review	Date performed

History in last year of   Admission for hyperglycaemia
Hypoglycaemia requiring professional attention
Anginal/myocardial infarction
Transient ischaemic attack/stroke

Claudication/amputation: above or below ankle

Erectile impotence

Procedures undertaken	Date performed	Result

Body mass index

Urinalysis for proteinuria/microalbuminuria

Blood pressure: systolic and diastolic

Tobacco consumption (cigarettes/day)

Glycated haemoglobin (or fructosamine)

Serum cholesterol and triglycerides

Serum creatinine

Visual acuity and ophthalmoscopy for cataract and retinopathy

Foot examination for pulses, vibration sensation and ulceration and general care

Diabetes therapy: insulin/oral hypoglycaemic agents/diet only

Hypertension and hyperlipidaemia therapy

Review by dietitian and/or chiropodist in last year

Routine follow-up:	GP only
	Shared care
	Hospital only

Chronic disease management – diabetes programme

Annual report

An annual report on the diabetes programme must be submitted. The following information may be requested – not all Health Authorities require all this information, although practices must be prepared to provide it if asked:

- Confirmation that a *register of all diabetic patients in the practice* is in place and that it is regularly updated.
- Confirmation that the *clinical management programme* has proceeded as planned, that patients are being offered regular reviews and that call and recall systems are in place.

- Confirmation that all *practice nurses contributing to the programme have been appropriately trained,* giving names and details of courses in diabetes management attended.
- Confirmation that *attached staff* have contributed to the programme as envisaged (with details).
- Confirmation that *records have been kept as planned* and, if not, that details of changes have been made during the year.
- A *summary of any audit activities* undertaken in the programme area.
- *Additional information* regarding any activities in the programme area other than those originally submitted (with details).
- Completion of a *statistical return* regarding numbers, age, sex, and whether type 1 or type 2 diabetes.
- Completion of *statistical return regarding number of annual reviews* (type 1 and type 2 diabetes) carried out in hospital, shared care or by the practice alone.

Guidelines are supplied by the Health Authority for the completion of the in-year monitoring return and annual report.

Further reading

Audit Commission (2000). *Testing Times: A review of diabetes services in England and Wales.* London: Audit Commission.

British Diabetic Association. Diabetes Services Advisory Committee (1993). *Recommendations for the Management of Diabetes in Primary Care: A revision of recommendations for diabetes health promotion clinics.* London: BDA.

Kenny C (1997). The use of computers in primary diabetes care. *Practical Diabetes International* **14**: 132–3.

Marks L (1996). *Counting the Cost: The real impact of non-insulin-dependent diabetes.* London: King's Fund/BDA.

Part III

About diabetes

16

Diabetes mellitus: a history of the condition

- Classification and types
- History

Diabetes is a wonderful affection, not very frequent among men, being a melting down of the flesh and limbs into urine . . . life is short, disgusting and painful, thirst unquenchable, death inevitable.

Aretaeus, the Cappadocian (AD 2)

Classification and types

Diabetes mellitus is a complex, metabolic disease characterised by high blood glucose concentrations. It is associated with impaired insulin production and/or action, resulting in the body's inability to utilise nutrients properly. It is believed that various genetic and environmental or lifestyle factors influence the cause and prognosis of the condition. Important differences in the frequency of diabetes and its complications have been reported between countries, ethnic and cultural groups.

It has never been easy to classify and diagnose diabetes mellitus, because its very heterogeneity and characteristics have rendered most attempts at subdivision not entirely accurate and unable to reflect its underlying nature. There were anomalies in the earliest classification by age of onset and the replacement by pathogenic mechanism (type 1 diabetes, type 2 diabetes, IGT, IFG), which was linked to treatment, also caused confusion and uncertainty. New diagnostic criteria set by the WHO were ratified in 2000.

The recommendation made by the World Health Organization (WHO) in 2000 defined IGT as a fasting glucose of < 7.0 mmol/l and an OGGT 2-hour value of ≥ 7.8 mmol/ but < 11.1 mmol/l.

At the present time, the major clinical classes of glucose intolerance include type 1 and type 2 diabetes mellitus, malnutrition-related diabetes mellitus (MRDM), impaired glucose tolerance (IGT), impaired fasting glycaemia (IFG) and gestational diabetes (which includes gestational IGT and gestational diabetes mellitus or GDM). Terms and definitions used to describe and diagnose diabetes were unified and adopted in 1979–80, updated in 1985, reflecting the tenth revision of the *International Classification of Diseases and Health-related Problems* (ICD-10), and new ones were added by the WHO in 2000.

History

Diabetes has been known and recognised for many thousands of years as a disease characterised by weakness, thirst and frequency of micturition. Aretaeus, a contemporary of Galen, noted that the Greek word for a siphon had been given to diabetes because 'the fluid does not remain in the body, but uses the body as a ladder, whereby to leave it!'.

Early treatments are described in the Ebers Papyrus written around 1500 BC, found in a grave in Thebes in Egypt in 1862. The treatment, 'to drive away the passing of too much urine . . .' described a medicine including a mixture of bones, wheat grains, fresh fruits, green lead, earth and water. These ingredients the user should 'let stand moist, strain it, take it for 4 days'.

In modern times, the sweet taste of urine passed by people with this disease was noted by Willis in the late seventeenth century and Matthew Dobson of Liverpool demonstrated that the sweet taste was caused by sugar. The Latin word for honeysweet *'mellitus'* was added to distinguish the disease from diabetes insipidus, a pituitary disorder, in which a large volume of sugar-free urine is passed.

In 1815 the French chemist, Chevraul, showed that the sugar in diabetic urine was glucose. The association between diabetes and the pancreas was not recognised until much later. Paul Langerhans described the pancreatic islet cells in the mid-nineteenth century and, in 1889, Mering and Minkowski produced fatal diabetes by removing the pancreas in animals.

The real breakthrough came in 1921–22, when in Toronto Frederick Banting and Charles Best discovered insulin:

> Those who watched the first starved, sometimes comatose diabetics receive insulin and return to life saw one of the genuine miracles of modern medicine. They were present at the closest approach to the resurrection of the body that our secular society can achieve and at the discovery of what has become the elixir of life for millions of human beings around the world.

So wrote Michael Bliss, the Canadian historian, in his definitive work on the discovery of insulin. Further research, however, revealed the complex physiology involved in the aetiology of the disease and in the development of complications. It was recognised that there were a number of different forms of diabetes. The discovery of insulin marked the therapeutic period. It confirmed the concept of a deficiency of insulin action as the basic abnormality in diabetes and gave rise to the differentiation between type 1 diabetes mellitus and non-type 2 diabetes mellitus.

Pharmaceutical research and development relating to type 1 diabetes has concentrated on developing 'purer' and more effective forms of insulin and new methods of delivery by 'pens' and 'pumps', although the latter have failed to live up to their early promise. Recombinant technology developed during the 1980s dramatically changed the availability and use of insulin. Animal insulin was no longer the sole source of the hormone. Insulin could now be produced in unlimited quantities of a purity close to 'human' insulin. This technology enabled the genetic blueprint of porcine insulin to be altered to produce an alternative insulin, close to the human species.

Oral hypoglycaemic agents were first introduced in Germany in 1955 and have been extensively developed. There are four main groups, the sulphonyl-ureas, the biguanides, thiazolidinediones and postprandial glucose regulators (PPGRs). The sulphonylureas act mainly by stimulating the release of insulin from the β cells in the pancreas. The action of the biguanide group is less clear but is believed to increase the peripheral uptake of glucose. The thiazolidine-diones reduce blood glucose and insulin levels by reducing insulin resistance. The PPGRs have a similar mode of action to sulphonylureas but with a faster onset and shorter duration.

Diet is the 'cornerstone' of treatment. An interesting observation on the effect of food on the incidence and progression of diabetes was made by the French physician Bouchardat in 1875, during the Prussian siege of Paris. The siege was prolonged and as food supplies ran out, forcing the population to eat cats and dogs, he noticed the absence of new cases in his practice and an improvement in the condition of those already diagnosed. Similar observations were made in the two world wars when national death rates for diabetes noticeably fell.

Dietary recommendations have changed from a restricted carbohydrate intake to a regimen low in fat and high in unrefined carbohydrates and dietary fibre. For the overweight, reduction in energy intake remains the most important aim. Carbohydrate should make up about 50–55% of the energy intake, preferably from foods naturally high in dietary fibre. Up to 25 g of added sucrose per day may be allowed, provided it is part of a diet low in fat and high in fibre.

Dietary advice in the treatment of diabetes is not only aimed at the control of blood glucose but also at the prevention of cardiovascular disease. In general it is the same advice as that offered to the general population.

The discovery of insulin by Banting and Best highlighted and accelerated the quest for understanding of the condition. As more has become known, the search for the causes of diabetes has moved towards further study of the immune system, the role of infection and the genetic implications already identified.

Further reading

Besser GM, Bodansky HI, Cudworth AG (1988). *Clinical Diabetes – An Illustrated Text.* Oxford: Gower Medical Publishing.

Bliss M (1983). *The Discovery of Insulin.* London: Macmillan Press.

British Diabetic Association Report (1992). Dietary recommendations for people with diabetes. *Diabetic Medicine* 9:189–202.

Day J (1998). *Living with Diabetes: The BDA guide for those treated with diet and tablets.* Chichester: John Wiley & Sons.

Laing W, Williams R (1989). *Diabetes: a model for health care management.* Office of Health Economics.

17   Type 1 diabetes mellitus

Formerly termed 'acute diabetes' or 'juvenile-onset diabetes', this type commonly occurs in childhood, adolescence and on into adult life. Symptoms of profound weight loss, excessive thirst, polyuria, lethargy and occasionally abdominal pain require immediate treatment with insulin. Should treatment not be available, ketoacidosis, coma and death are inevitable. The onset is sudden (days or weeks).

Diagnosis

Diagnosis is usually straightforward, based on the presenting symptoms and raised blood glucose levels (> 11.1 mmol/l venous plasma or > 12.2 mmol/l capillary plasma). After diagnosis, insulin therapy is started together with appropriate family support and education about living with diabetes in all its aspects. Discussion about modification of food intake and activity in relation to the person's life is staged alongside the stabilisation process. A careful multidisciplinary approach with empathy and consistent, correct advice is vital in fostering a healthy 'life with insulin' and in the reduction of acute and long-term complications.

Two acute complications (hypoglycaemia and hyperglycaemia) occur in relation to insulin therapy and are associated with the extremes of blood glucose levels.

Hypoglycaemia

Hypoglycaemia (blood glucose levels < 4 mmol/l) may occur with little warning, as a result of too much insulin, insufficient food, delayed meals, alcohol, extra activity or stress.

Hyperglycaemia

Hyperglycaemia (blood glucose levels > 10 mmol/l, progressing to higher levels) is the second acute complication of insulin therapy. Vomiting, dehydration and ketosis will develop into severe fluid depletion, disordered blood chemistry and electrolyte imbalance which, if uncorrected, may be irreversible and death will follow. The situation occurs during illness or may occur where the psychological state is severely affected resulting in the person using insulin as a tool of manipulation.

Improved support services and the development of technology allowing people with diabetes the opportunity to check their own blood glucose levels have, over many years, now greatly improved their confidence in the self-management of their insulin therapy and in the prevention of occasions of 'acute complications'. This self-regulation of blood glucose is particularly important during pregnancy, where strict blood glucose control is vital even before conception. Pre-pregnancy counselling and blood glucose levels between 4 mmol/l and 7 mmol/l are essential to avoid fetal abnormality or death. Thirty years ago, about one-quarter of pregnancies in women with diabetes ended in fetal death. Now almost all are successful. This improvement is the result of major developments in obstetric, diabetic and paediatric care. Major congenital abnormalities, however, still occur more frequently than in non-diabetic pregnancies.

The causes of type 1 diabetes

Factors involved in the causation of type 1 diabetes are complex. Genetic factors are not only involved but also environmental factors, demonstrated by changes in islet cells and destruction of β cells, either directly or by triggering an autoimmune response. Possible environmental agents suggested are infective conditions (perhaps occurring some years before) as well as physical, chemical and psychological factors.

The prevalence of type 1 diabetes varies considerably in different countries, based on estimates, varying levels of ascertainment and population age structure. Prevalence appears to be higher further from the Equator, in particular in Scandinavia, and lower than average in Japan.

Seasonal variations in incidence are also of interest as they are consistent and occur all over the world. Higher incidence rates are reported during the autumn and winter months than over the spring and summer periods. Seasonal variations are thought to be associated with the presence of infective agents such as viruses. These may trigger the onset of the disease in susceptible people, in particular young people where incidence is age related and peaks around the ages of 5 and 12 years, coinciding with changes of school environments and the onset of puberty.

SUMMARY

- The prevalence of type 1 diabetes is about one-tenth that of type 2 diabetes in Western communities.
- Clinical onset occurs during childhood particularly around the time of puberty.
- The condition also appears in early and later adulthood.
- There is a higher incidence in autumn and winter and an increasing gradient in incidence from southern to northern latitudes.

Further reading

Bramer GR (1988). *International Statistical Classification of Disease and Health-related Problems* – Tenth Revision. *World Health Statistics Quarterly* **41**: 32–6.

Day J (1998). *Living with Diabetes: The BDA guide for those treated with insulin*. Chichester: John Wiley & Sons.

Laing W, Williams R (1989). *Diabetes: a model for health care management*. Office of Health Economics.

Pyke DA, Nelson PE (1976). Diabetes mellitus in identical twins. In: *The Genetics of Diabetes Mellitus* (Crevtzfeldt W, Kobbenking I, Neel JV, eds). Berlin: Springer Verlag, 194–202.

Rewers M et al. (1988). Trends in the prevalence and incidence of diabetes. Insulin dependent diabetes in childhood. *World Health Statistics Quarterly* **41**: 179–89.

Watkins PI (1988). *ABC of Diabetes*. London: BMJ Publishing.

WHO Technical Report Series No 727 (1985). *Diabetes Mellitus. Report of a WHO Study Group*. Geneva: WHO.

17

18 Type 2 diabetes mellitus

Type 2 diabetes mellitus, the most common form of diabetes, increases in prevalence from 30–35 years of age. By 70 years of age, prevalence is usually three to four times higher than the overall prevalence in adults (2–5% in European and North American communities). *Undiagnosed* type 2 diabetes has been reported in almost equal proportions to diagnosed diabetes in many societies.

In developing countries, type 2 diabetes is rare in the traditional setting but has become very common, exceeding 1%, in adults in many urbanised communities. Several ethnic groups have a greater genetic predisposition to type 2 diabetes than do white people. In the absence of effective interventions, the prevalence of type 2 diabetes in all populations is likely to rise, as a result of ageing, a reduction in infectious disease mortality and increases in the prevalence of obesity, lack of regular physical exercise and inappropriate diet.

Efforts to prevent obesity through diet alone have been generally unsuccessful. Physical activity, however, appears to have an important role in the prevention of type 2 diabetes through its association with reduced body weight and through independent effects on insulin resistance and glucose tolerance. Further research is needed to assess the magnitude of the benefits of exercise and to determine the most effective exercise programmes for reducing the incidence of type 2 diabetes. To date, research has failed to demonstrate an association between type 2 diabetes and specific genetic markers even though it is a familial disease.

Both sexes are affected in type 2 diabetes, although in some communities a male preponderance is shown, for example, in India and in Asian Indians in the UK. In other communities, females make up most of those with the disease. In populations where type 2 diabetes is common, it may be encountered in adolescence and among young adults. This form of diabetes, which has a familial distribution compatible with a dominant mode of inheritance, is sometimes referred to as mature-onset diabetes of the young (MODY).

Diagnosis

The diagnosis of type 2 diabetes is less clear cut than that of type 1 (Table 18.1). Hitherto, the condition has been called 'mild' diabetes of maturity onset; it is rare below the age of 35 years (when it is likely to be wrongly termed MODY). The onset is insidious and may be revealed only at routine screening. Symptoms of lethargy, thirst and polyuria are the most common but may proceed unnoticed until an episode of stress or an infection precipitates the severity of symptoms, forcing the individual to seek help. The diagnosis will be established by raised blood glucose levels (venous blood $\geq$ 7.0 mmol/l fasting or random levels of $\geq$ 11.1 mmol/l).

Table 18.1 Differences between type 1 and type 2 diabetes

	Type 1 diabetes	Type 2 diabetes
Proportions (%)	10–20	80–90
Usual age of onset (years)	< 40	> 40
Speed of onset	Rapid	Gradual
Likelihood of ketosis	High	Low
Complications at presentation	No	Yes, frequently
Treatment	Diet and insulin	Diet alone, diet and tablets, or diet and insulin
Likelihood of hypoglycaemia	More	Less but dangerous in elderly people
Precipitated by obesity	No	Yes
Majority of care provision	Hospital	General practitioner

Should blood glucose levels be raised but less than these values, a glucose tolerance test should be performed by the patient taking 75 g of glucose under specified conditions and, after a measurement of a fasting blood glucose level, sequential blood glucose levels are then tested. The results are interpreted according to WHO criteria to confirm the presence or absence of diabetes or the existence of impaired glucose tolerance. A new value has been added into the WHO criteria (2000) – IFG (fasting plasma glucose $\geq$ 6.1 mmol/l, < 7.0 mmol/l).

Treatment

Treatment for people with type 2 diabetes is aimed at the alleviation of symptoms, the reduction of blood glucose levels and, where possible, the prevention of complications. Should the patient be overweight the first line of treatment consists of dietary modification and education to reduce weight. If successful, this may lead to a reduction in blood glucose levels and symptomatic relief.

Should this line of treatment be unsuccessful, oral hypoglycaemic agents may be required. Should these fail to achieve the desired result, insulin therapy may be required. The normal weight or underweight person unable to obtain symptom relief and/or reduction in blood glucose levels with dietary modification and hypoglycaemic agents will usually require insulin sooner rather than later.

Extreme caution is required in treatment with oral hypoglycaemic agents (and insulin therapy) in elderly people, to avoid the complication of hypoglycaemia. People with type 2 diabetes may require insulin in the short term in times of illness or during a surgical intervention. The complications of insulin treatment in type 2 diabetes are those of hypoglycaemia and weight gain. The problem of hypoglycaemia often deters the instigation of this therapy. A short-term 'trial' of insulin may provide the answer as to the best course of treatment.

Combined regimens of oral hypoglycaemic agents (sulphonylureas) and insulin have been used in some centres but to little advantage. The livelihood of people with diabetes must also be considered. People holding particular types of driving licences such as Large Goods Vehicle (LGV) and Passenger-Carrying Vehicle (PCV) will lose these should insulin therapy be instituted. A most difficult problem to be solved occurs when insulin is used in the treatment of symptomless people with type 2 diabetes, where weight gain progresses with no improvement in blood glucose levels.

18

SUMMARY

■ Type 2 diabetes is common, affecting 2–5% of the population, rising with age.
■ The onset usually occurs after the age of 35 years.
■ Type 2 diabetes is not a 'mild condition'. It is associated with considerable morbidity and mortality.
■ Weight gain and physical inactivity are important factors in the progression of the condition.
■ Treatment is complex, particularly in older people.

Further reading

Alberti KGMM (1991). The diagnosis and classification of diabetes mellitus. *Diabetes Voice* 44: 35–41.

Besser GM, Bodansky HJ, Cudworth AG (1988). *Clinical Diabetes – An Illustrated Text.* London: Gower Medical Publishing.

British Diabetic Association (1988). *Diabetes in the United Kingdom.* London: BDA.

Day J (1998). *Living with Diabetes: The BDA guide for those treated with diet and tablets.* Chichester: John Wiley & Sons.

Diabetes UK (2000). *New Diagnostic Criteria for Diabetes: Summary of changes.* Factsheet. London: Diabetes UK.

Harris MI (1987). Prevalence of diabetes and impaired glucose tolerance in US population aged 20–74 years. *Diabetes* 36:523–34.

Manson JE et al. (1991). Physical activity and incidence of non-insulin-dependent diabetes in women. *Lancet* 338:774–8.

O'Rahilly S et al. (1988). Type II (non-insulin-dependent diabetes mellitus). New genetics for old nightmares. *Diabetologia* 31:407–14.

Peacock I, Tattersall RB (1984). The difficult choice of treatment for poorly controlled maturity onset diabetes: tablets or insulin? *British Medical Journal* 288:1956–9.

Rudermann M, Apelian AZ, Schneider SM (1990). Exercise in therapy and prevention of type II diabetes: implications for blacks. *Diabetes Care* 13(suppl 4): 1163–8.

World Health Organization (2000). *Definition, Diagnosis and Classification of Diabetes Mellitus and its Complications.* Geneva: WHO.

19 Other categories of diabetes (as defined by WHO)

Impaired glucose tolerance

The US National Diabetes Data Group introduced the category of impaired glucose tolerance (IGT) in 1979 and this was later endorsed by the WHO Expert Committee Report No 646 in 1980. The recommendations made by the WHO in 2000 define IGT as a fasting plasma glucose of < 7.0 mmol/l and an OGTT 2-hour value of ≥ 7.8 mmol/l but < 11.1 mmol/l.

Previously, the term 'borderline' diabetes had been used to distinguish between people whose glucose tolerance was 'impaired' in relation to the non-diabetic population but who were not frankly diabetic. The IGT category removed the label of 'diabetes' because this level of glucose intolerance is not associated with the development of microvascular complications.

Impaired glucose tolerance is, however, associated with increased risk of death from ischaemic heart disease. A proportion of people with IGT progress to diabetes within a few years. Estimates range from 1% to 5% depending on age and subsequent duration of follow-up.

Impaired fasting glycaemia

This category was introduced by the WHO to classify individuals who have fasting glucose values above the normal range, but below those diagnostic of diabetes. The fasting plasma glucose is ≥ 6.1 mmol/l but < 7.0 mmol/l.

Diabetes UK recommends that all those who have impaired fasting glycaemia (IFG) should have an OGGT to exclude the diagnosis of diabetes; they are actively managed with lifestyle advice. If the glucose remains elevated above

6 mmol/l after at least 3 months, treatment with an oral hypoglycaemic agent should be considered in the light of the findings of UKPDS.

It should be noted that IGT and IFG are not clinical entities in their own right, but risk categories for cardiovascular disease (IGT) and/or future diabetes (IFG).

Gestational diabetes mellitus

Gestational diabetes is defined as carbohydrate intolerance of variable severity with onset or first recognition during the present pregnancy. The definition applies, whether insulin is used for treatment or the condition persists after pregnancy, but does not exclude the possibility that the glucose intolerance may have antedated the pregnancy. This abnormal glucose intolerance is generally indicated by a fasting venous blood glucose concentration of 6 mmol/l or above. It is extremely unlikely that such a fasting level would occur in a non-diabetic woman. A fasting level of 6 mmol/l or above is associated with increased morbidity in the fetus.

Gestational diabetes has been retained as a term by the new WHO diagnostic criteria, but it now encompasses the group formerly classified as gestational impaired glucose intolerance (GIGT) and gestational diabetes mellitus (GDM). Diabetes UK endorses the use of the WHO definition to allow for comparative studies. As glucose tolerance changes with the duration of pregnancy, however, the gestation at which the diagnosis was made should be recorded and, if made in the third trimester, the doctor should be cautious about the clinical implication of IGT. Some concern has been expressed that the WHO level is too tight for everyday clinical practice, and the Diabetes Care Advisory Committee is currently consulting on revised recommendations. Until these are published clinicians should use their own clinical judgement when diagnosing gestational diabetes. There is a very high risk of GDM in subsequent pregnancies.

Generally, gestational diabetes resolves post partum. The condition includes those with a genetic or acquired susceptibility, in whom the metabolic changes of pregnancy induce a temporary diabetic state. People with a 'low level' of diabetes present before pregnancy, become symptomatic and are diagnosed at routine screening during antenatal care.

It is important that women at risk of developing gestational diabetes are identified, because the condition is associated with an increased incidence of perinatal morbidity and the development of diabetes by the mother in later life.

Antenatal care should include the following assessment:

■ Previous gestational diabetes or IGT or IFG
■ Family history of diabetes

- Maternal obesity (>120% ideal body weight)
- Previous delivery of a large baby
- Previous unexplained still birth
- Certain ethnic groups (Indo-Pakistani women in central London have an 8.6% incidence of an abnormal glucose tolerance test)
- Women over 25 years of age
- Previous obstetric and/or perinatal complications
- Recurrent urinary tract infections or candidiasis.

Once the history is known, those 'at risk' are identified for testing. Owing to the low renal threshold that exists in pregnancy, urine testing is of little value. Overt diabetes is missed and only a few of those with impaired glucose tolerance are identified. A full oral glucose tolerance test is impractical for screening the antenatal population, although it is the only definitive test for the diagnosis of gestational diabetes.

The management of gestational diabetes involves intensive team work between obstetric and diabetes carers and involves support for the woman throughout pregnancy. Tight blood glucose control with dietary modification and/or insulin therapy is required, similar to a pregnant woman with established diabetes, to avoid antenatal complications and perinatal morbidity and mortality. Oral hypoglycaemic agents are not used in the treatment of gestational diabetes or diabetes in pregnancy. Particular support is required for women with gestational diabetes when they are first diagnosed in order that treatment can be commenced quickly and blood glucose levels lowered as soon as possible. Obstetric management is similar to that provided for women with diabetes.

After delivery, a full oral glucose tolerance test is performed 6–8 weeks post partum. Advice is given regarding the maintenance of ideal body weight and that gestational diabetes may recur in subsequent pregnancies. Should the glucose tolerance test be abnormal, referral to a diabetes team for follow-up is required and treatment, support and further education provided.

It is generally accepted that 40% of women with gestational diabetes will develop type 2 diabetes within 20 years. This is usually type 2. An awareness of this is important in the avoidance of long-term complications of diabetes.

19

Further reading

Alberti KGMM (1991). The diagnosis and classification of diabetes mellitus. *Diabetes Voice* **44**: 35–41.

Beard RW, Moet IJ (1982). Is gestational diabetes a clinical entity? *Diabetologia* **23**: 307–12.

Chahal P (1988). *Diabetes and Pregnancy.* London: Butterworths.

Oakley CE (1992). Care of gestational diabetes. *Diabetes Care* **1**: 6–8.

World Health Organization (2000). *Definition, Diagnosis and classification of Diabetes Mellitus and its Complications.* Geneva: WHO.

Other causes of diabetes – secondary diabetes

- Hormonal causes of diabetes
- Pancreatic disease
- Haemochromatosis
- Drug-induced diabetes
- Tumours of the islet cells
- Hereditary causes
- Malnutrition-related diabetes mellitus

There are many disorders or syndromes associated with secondary diabetes. Relatively, however, they account for a small number of patients with the condition.

Hormonal causes of diabetes

Overt diabetes or glucose intolerance is often associated with Cushing's syndrome. If the causative tumour is removed or the Cushing's syndrome treated, the diabetes can be improved or even cured.

About a third of patients with acromegaly develop diabetes which improves on treatment of the acromegalic condition. Phaeochromocytoma also produces glucose intolerance which may be intermittent.

Patients with tumours producing corticosteroids, ACTH, growth hormone, glucagon and catecholamines all induce insulin resistance.

Pancreatic disease

Severe disease of the pancreas or pancreatectomy causes diabetes which may require insulin therapy. As glucagon is absent after these pancreatic conditions, control of the diabetes is erratic and may require only small doses of insulin –

or severe hypoglycaemia results. Acute pancreatitis, cystic fibrosis and chronic pancreatitis may cause diabetes.

Carcinoma of the pancreas

The appearance of diabetes and jaundice almost simultaneously, usually within a few weeks, suggests the diagnosis of this condition. When surgery is indicated, insulin therapy will almost always be required.

Haemochromatosis

A condition of defective iron metabolism results in the accumulation of iron in the tissues and over-absorption of iron which may result in the concentration of iron in the liver and pancreas to 50–100 times normal levels. Other endocrine glands show heavy iron deposits. Patients with this condition are usually male, aged 40–60 years, with a ratio of 9:1 (males:females). Two-thirds of people with haemochromatosis have diabetes, usually requiring insulin.

Drug-induced diabetes

Thiazides reduce glucose tolerance by impairing insulin secretion. Thiazide diuretics may have a significant hyperglycaemic effect in type 2 diabetes.

Corticosteroids impair glucose tolerance mainly by increasing glucose production and increasing insulin resistance. Diabetic control is worsened by corticosteroids soon after administration. These drugs may precipitate diabetes; they do not cause the condition unless large doses are used, as in transplant therapy, to counter rejection episodes. Diabetes is most likely to occur in people who have had impaired glucose tolerance or gestational diabetes. Thyroxine may impair glucose tolerance although not sufficiently to alter diabetic control. The combined oestrogen–progestogen contraceptive pill only mildly impairs glucose tolerance and does not affect diabetic control in type 1 diabetes.

Tumours of the islet cells

Glucagonoma is a rare tumour of the islet-secreting A cells, producing characteristic clinical features, skin rashes, anaemia, thromboembolic disease and diabetes. A very rare tumour is a somatostatinoma of the D cells and is commonly associated with diabetes.

Insulinomas are tumours of the islet cells containing large amounts of insulin; they cause hypoglycaemia in people who do not have diabetes. Surgical removal of the tumour usually cures this condition.

Hereditary causes

There are around 50 genetic syndromes associated with clinical diabetes or impaired glucose tolerance. These, however, are rare. Examples of well documented genetic syndromes are:

■ **DIDMOAD syndrome** (**d**iabetes **i**nsipidus, **d**iabetes **m**ellitus, **o**ptic **a**trophy and **d**eafness) is maternally inherited and type 1 diabetes is associated with the development of diabetes insipidus, blindness from optic atrophy and gradual onset of high tone deafness.
■ **Mature-onset of diabetes in the young (MODY)** is also known as Mason's syndrome and follows a pattern of dominant inheritance. Occurring in the young, the person affected remains non-insulin requiring for many years. (The term 'Mason' relates to the first family in whom the syndrome was recognised.)

Other disorders associated with secondary diabetes are Addison's disease (more common in people with type 1 diabetes than in the general population), hypopituitarism and thyroid disease.

Malnutrition-related diabetes mellitus (MRDM)

A significant proportion of younger people (onset usually below 30 years of age) in tropical developing countries do not fall into either of the two main classes of diabetes (type 1 and type 2 diabetes). These people have a particular set of symptoms and metabolic types to justify special categorisation. Malnutrition-related diabetes may constitute 30–60% of all cases of young-onset diabetes in developing countries.

20

SUMMARY

Secondary causes of diabetes

■ Hormonal
■ Pancreatic disease
■ Carcinoma of the pancreas
■ Haemochromatosis
■ Drug induced – especially steroids and thiazides
■ Tumours of the islet cells
■ Hereditary causes
■ Malnutrition-related diabetes (seen in developing countries)

Further reading

Bajaj JS (ed.) (1984). Malnutrition related diabetes. In: *Diabetes Mellitus in Developing Countries.* New Delhi: Interprint Publishers.

Bajaj JS, Subbaro B (1988). Malnutrition related diabetes mellitus. In: *World Book of Diabetes in Practice,* Vol. 3. Oxford: Elsevier Science Publishers BV (Biomedical Division), p. 25.

Laing W, Williams R (1989). *Diabetes: a Model for Health Care Management.* Office of Health Economics.

Siddle NC, Knight MA (1991). *Managing the Menopause. A Practical Guide to HRT.* Oxted: Medical Communications Services.

Watkins PJ, Drury PL, Howell SL (1996). *Diabetes and its Management,* 5th edn. Oxford: Blackwell Science.

21 The complications of diabetes

■ Some specific complications
■ Increased frequency of other diseases
■ Aspirin treatment in diabetes

Two important factors in the causation of complications of diabetes are:

1. Hyperglycaemia
2. The duration of diabetes.

The long-term complications of type 1 diabetes, those of nephropathy, retinopathy, autonomic and peripheral neuropathy are rarely seen before 5–7 years' duration of the condition. Most commonly, they do not occur before 10–20 years. In type 2 diabetes, however, complications may be present at diagnosis, the condition having been unrecognised for several years before presentation. As duration of diabetes lengthens, complications may progress, although, after 30 years' duration, the annual incidence decreases. Some people with diabetes of 30–60 years' duration are free from the long-term complications of the condition.

Other factors in the development of complications are vascular changes which are affected by metabolic dysfunction. Genetic markers of susceptibility have not been identified. The eyes, the kidneys and the peripheral nerves are the organs most affected by diabetes. These organs may be affected to a different extent, one being severely affected while another is not damaged at all. The 'hallmark' of long-standing diabetes is the thickening of basement membrane which can be observed in the kidney, retina, nerves, skin, muscle and adipose tissue. Biochemical dysfunction is also identified as a possible problem in relation to the glycosylation of proteins and pathways of sorbitol. Associations exist between the major complications of diabetes, with patterns of association more marked in type 1 diabetes (such as retinopathy, nephropathy and neuropathy in the same person) than in type 2 diabetes.

21

SUMMARY

Major complications of diabetes
Specific

1. Renal disease   Diabetic nephropathy

2. Eye disease   Background retinopathy
                                    Diabetic maculopathy
                                    Proliferative retinopathy

3. Neuropathy   Autonomic neuropathy
                                    Peripheral neuropathy
                                    Cranial nerve palsies
                                    Peripheral mononeuropathy
                                    Diabetic amyotrophy

Increased frequency of other diseases

1. Cardiac problems   Coronary heart disease

2. Eyes   Cataracts

Some specific complications

Renal disease – diabetic nephropathy

Diabetic nephropathy is recognised as a major cause of morbidity and mortality in people with type 1 diabetes affecting some 40% of patients developing the disease before the age of 31 years. Reliable information regarding nephropathy in people with type 2 diabetes is less available, as precise identification of the onset of this condition is difficult to ascertain. However, the relative risk of death from renal failure in this group is thought to be lower in older patients. The problem is still a major one in terms of prevalence because 75–90% of people with diabetes have type 2. It is reported that between 32% and 90% of this large group enter treatment programmes for end-stage renal disease.

Next to glomerulonephritis, diabetes is ranked as the most common cause for patients requiring renal dialysis and transplantation. A specific type of renal lesion occurs in the glomerular capillaries known as diabetic glomerulo-sclerosis. Diabetic renal failure and its progression can be described in four stages.

Stage 1

At initial diagnosis of type 1 diabetes, there may be an elevated glomerular filtration rate as high as 160 ml/min (normal levels 120 ml/min). This is known as hyperfiltration. This abnormality may be reversible with insulin treatment over a period of weeks or months. However, a normal glomerular filtration rate is usually never achieved. The patient is said to hyperfiltrate continually leading in the long term to structural damage in the glomerulus.

Stage 2

Taking on average 10–15 years to reach this stage, damaged glomeruli allow the passage of clinically undetectable amounts of protein to be filtered into the urine. This is termed 'microalbuminuria'. The importance of lower concentrations of albumin excretion has been recognised in recent years. Microalbuminuria has been applied to an albumin excretion rate of 30–300 mg/day. This level of increased albumin excretion would not be identified on standard dipstick testing for proteinuria (e.g. with Albustix or Uristix) but has been shown in patients with type 1 diabetes to be highly predictive of progression to overt nephropathy and renal failure. In type 2 diabetes, studies have suggested a prevalence of microalbuminuria of 12–16%. The prevalence of this condition is higher in certain ethnic groups. It is more common in people from the Indian subcontinent than in white people in the UK.

Microalbuminuria can now be detected using stick tests (e.g. from Roche Diagnostics). Regular animal testing for microalbuminuria has been demonstrated to be both sensitive and specific in the detection of early renal disease in type 1 diabetes. The use of this test is also of importance in the early indication of large-vessel disease and diabetic retinopathy in type 1 diabetes. Testing for microalbuminuria in type 2 diabetes is not at present in widespread use. This may enter into clinical practice once there is research evidence that the text is sensitive and specific, and provides indicators for complications and early intervention in type 2 diabetes.

Stage 3

Overt diabetic renal failure is present at this stage. Proteinuria can be detected by Albustix testing. Severe proteinuria presents as nephrotic syndrome. At this stage, the glomerular filtration rate starts to decline with rising serum urea and creatinine levels, indicating diabetic renal failure.

21

Stage 4

Finally, the glomerular filtration rate is no longer able to maintain haemostasis, resulting in end-stage renal failure, requiring dialysis or renal transplantation.

Delaying the progression of diabetic nephropathy

There are three main elements of treatment involved in the delay of the progression of diabetic nephropathy.

Detection and control of raised blood pressure

Detection and control of raised blood pressure by aggressive hypertensive treatment postpone renal insufficiency in diabetic nephropathy.

Glycaemic control

If this is achieved in the early stages of the condition, albumin excretion may be reduced. There is early evidence that early use of angiotensin-converting enzyme (ACE) inhibitors can retard the development of nephropathy and retinopathy.

Protein restriction in the diet (in type 1 diabetes)

This may have a beneficial effect on microalbuminuria, independent of changes in glucose concentrations and arterial blood pressure. The patient should be seen by a dietitian to assess the diet and recommend appropriate changes.

Once renal failure is established haemodialysis, continuous ambulatory peritoneal dialysis (CAPD) and renal transplantation are the only options available for the continuation of life.

Tests for microalbuminuria

Micral Test urine strips
Roche Diagnostics Ltd
Bell Lane
Lewes
East Sussex
BN7 1LG
Tel: 01273 480444

SUMMARY

Diabetic nephropathy

- Affects 40% of people with type 1 diabetes diagnosed before the age of 31 years.
- Affects 32–90% of people with type 2 diabetes although figures less accurate as duration of type 2 may not be known.
- There are four stages of diabetic renal disease.
- Microalbuminuria may be detected at stage 2 after 10–15 years of diabetes.
- Microalbuminuria can be detected using simple tests.
- Raised serum urea and creatinine levels (stage 3) indicate renal failure.
- Delaying the progression of diabetic nephropathy involves three elements of treatment:
  - detection and control of raised blood pressure
  - glycaemic control
  - in type 1 diabetes, dietary protein restriction may be of benefit.
- Established renal failure will require the following treatment options:
  - haemodialysis
  - continuous ambulatory peritoneal dialysis (CAPD)
  - renal transplantation.

Eye disease – diabetic retinopathy

Diabetic retinopathy encompasses the retinovascular complications of diabetes. It is one of the major causes of blindness in developed countries. Two per cent of the population with diabetes have been estimated to be blind from diabetic retinopathy. In people under the age of 65 years, it is the most common cause of blindness, accounting for 19.7% of all new registrations in the 16–64 age group.

The incidence of diabetic retinopathy is closely related to the duration of diabetes and its progression is variable from slow to rapid onset. The frequency of diabetic retinopathy is increasing with the greater longevity of the diabetic population. It is estimated that, after 10 years of diabetic life, 20% will have diabetic retinopathy and, after 20 years, 80% of the diabetic population will be affected. L'Esperance estimated that 60% of people with diabetes with a duration of the disease for more than 15 years will have some form of retinopathy with females more commonly affected.

21

Diabetic retinopathy is rare in children, although it may occur, usually after the onset of puberty. This is thought to be the result of growth increase, hormonal changes and poor glycaemic control. As mentioned in the section on diabetic nephropathy, there is increasing evidence that early use of ACE inhibitors can retard development of retinopathy.

Background retinopathy

Microaneurysms, haemorrhages and yellow–white patches in rings (hard exudates) are characteristic and harmless, unless they occur on the macula (area of vision). Should the macula be oedematous, blindness may occur if this condition is not treated.

Proliferative retinopathy

Formation of 'new vessels' (pre-proliferative retinopathy) caused by retinal ischaemia is a dangerous sign and may proceed to proliferative retinopathy and haemorrhage, causing retinal detachment and other severe ocular disorders; these, in turn, lead to visual impairment and blindness.

Screening

For visual impairment and blindness to be averted, people with diabetes should be identified and screened (annually). Visual acuity should be checked at regular intervals, because deteriorating vision may indicate the presence of sight-threatening retinopathy, although normal visual acuity may occur even though retinopathy is present. After this test, examination of the fundi through dilated pupils should be carried out, to determine the presence or progress of retinopathy.

There is good evidence that improved patient education and regular screening programmes, combined with early detection of retinal changes and photocoagulation therapy, have major effects on reducing visual impairment and blindness in diabetes mellitus.

Effective treatment for diabetic retinopathy

Laser treatment is very effective at saving sight, particularly if carried out at an early stage of sight-threatening diabetic retinopathy. Severe visual loss relates to independent living, whereas moderate loss impacts on quality of life. This protection lasts for over 10 years in two-thirds of surviving laser-treated patients. Using data from epidemiological studies, each successful treatment will give at least 5 years of preserved sight.

SUMMARY

Diabetic retinopathy

- Diabetic retinopathy is one of the major causes of blindness in developed countries.
- It accounts for nearly 20% of blindness in the 16–64 age group.
- The incidence of retinopathy is related to the duration of diabetes.
- The onset of retinopathy may be rapid or slow.
- There are three main categories of diabetic retinopathy:
  - background retinopathy
  - pre-proliferative retinopathy
  - proliferative retinopathy.
- People with diabetes should be identified and their eyes screened annually.
- A screening programme should include testing for visual acuity and examination of the fundi through dilated pupils.
- Patient education, regular screening, early detection of retinal change and photocoagulation therapy reduce visual impairment and blindness.

Cataracts and diabetes mellitus

The association between cataracts and diabetes is well known. Cataracts may indicate the presence of diabetes and are more common in people with diabetes. It has also been shown that there is a significant association between the prevalence of cataract and age as well as duration of diabetes. This is important, because progression of this condition leading to severe visual impairment has profound implications on living with diabetes, quality of life and health care costs.

Diabetic neuropathy

Autonomic neuropathy

It is estimated that 20–40% of all people with diabetes have some abnormality of autonomic function. Insidious in onset, its presence may be undetected until late in its natural history. Dysfunction may be present in the cardiovascular system (causing postural hypotension), the alimentary tract (causing uncontrollable diarrhoea), the respiratory control system and in thermoregulation. Genitourinary disturbances are also distressing, one of the major problems being that of impotence. It has been reported that 50% of men with diabetes eventually become impotent. Few men attending diabetic clinics seek help and fewer are treated, although several effective treatments are now available.

Peripheral neuropathy

Almost 50% of people with diabetes have neuropathy affecting peripheral nerves, mainly those of the feet and legs. More hospital beds in Britain are occupied by patients who have diabetes and lower limb and foot problems than with all the other complications of diabetes combined. The two main features are neuropathy and ischaemia, often present together. Identification of those at risk of foot ulceration and preventive education are the most important aspects of the care of the neuropathic foot in the person with diabetes and in the prevention of prolonged hospital admission and amputation.

SUMMARY

Diabetic neuropathy

- Autonomic neuropathy affects 20–40% of all people with diabetes.
- Autonomic neuropathy may affect many body systems.
- Autonomic neuropathy causes impotence in 50% of men with diabetes. Treatment for this condition is available.
- Peripheral neuropathy affects 50% of people with diabetes.
- Lower limb and foot problems caused by peripheral neuropathy and ischaemia are common causing prolonged hospital admission and amputation.
- Identification of those at risk of foot ulceration and education are important preventive measures.

Increased frequency of other diseases

Type 2 diabetes: the metabolic syndrome

Also known as syndrome X and Reaven's syndrome, type 2 diabetes is a complex condition that is associated with:

- hypertension
- central obesity
- hyperlipidaemia
- hyperinsulinaemia
- polycystic ovary syndrome.

At the heart of this syndrome is the problem of insulin resistance. This is a vicious circle. Insulin resistance can lead to weight gain, which in turn worsens insulin resistance.

Insulin resistance

- Insulin resistance is one of the fundamental defects of type 2 diabetes.
- Insulin resistance is an early feature of the development of type 2 diabetes.
- The body fails to respond to its own insulin. This can initially be compensated for by an increase in insulin secretion.
- Insulin-resistant patients may become hyperinsulinaemic.
- Continued insulin resistance leads to the eventual exhaustion of the β cells. This results in a failure to produce adequate insulin and an increase in blood glucose.
- In type 2 diabetes, insulin resistance is characterised by: impaired (insulin-stimulated) glucose uptake by fat, liver and skeletal muscle, and over-production of glucose by the liver.
- Insulin resistance is central to the development of cardiovascular risk factors, which are clustered together in the metabolic syndrome described earlier.
- Regular vigorous exercise improves oxygen consumption and reduces insulin resistance, even in elderly people.
- The problems caused by insulin resistance can be reduced by lifestyle changes.
- Thiazolidinediones (also called PPAR-gamma agonists or glitazones) are new drugs that target insulin resistance. They improve glycaemic control by improving insulin sensitivity at key sites of insulin resistance – namely fat, liver and skeletal muscle.

Hypertension: treatment plans

- Raised blood pressure is very common in type 2 diabetes (40–50%).
- There is increasing evidence that aggressive BP treatment reduces vascular complications in diabetes.
- As a result, the threshold for starting treatment and the target for treatment are both falling.
- Start treatment if systolic BP > 150 or diastolic BP > 90 mmHg.
- Aim at normalising blood pressure (130/80), using HOT Study targets.
- Treat older people with equal enthusiasm, because they are more likely to derive early benefits.

21

- There is evidence that ACE (angiotensin-converting enzyme) inhibitors have a protective effect on kidneys in people with diabetes, and possibly reduce retinopathy over and above their effect in reducing blood pressure.
- The UKPDS (UK Prospective Diabetes Study) came up with the finding that ACE inhibitors confer no greater benefit than β blockers in hypertension. However, the UKPDS carries the simple messages:
  - high BP is common in type 2 diabetes
  - tight BP control has a major effect in reducing complications, including retinopathy
  - many patients need two or more drugs to achieve the target BP of 130/80.
- Doctors should continue using the antihypertensive drugs that they are familiar with, remembering that (in hypertension) compliance may be improved if a drug needs to be taken only once daily.
- All drugs used for treating hypertension have well-recognised side effects:
  - thiazides: low serum K^+, raised blood glucose and impotence
  - β blockers: may worsen asthma and peripheral vascular disease
  - ACE inhibitors: cough; in rare cases, they cause renal failure; angioneurotic oedema
  - calcium blockers: flushing, headache, oedema.

Cardiac disease and diabetes mellitus

Heart disease is a common cause of morbidity and mortality in people with diabetes. The Framingham study demonstrated that people with diabetes have increased morbidity and mortality from all cardiovascular causes which persist when the risk factors of hyperlipidaemia, hypertension and obesity are taken into account. The increased incidence of coronary artery disease in male and

---

Risk factors for coronary heart disease

- Increased concentrations of LDL-cholesterol
- Decreased concentrations of HDL-cholesterol
- Hyperglycaemia (HbA1c > 6.2%)
- Insulin resistance
- Hypertension
- Smoking
- Male sex

Suggestions for cholesterol screening in people with diabetes

- People with diabetes are at high risk of vascular disease and should be treated as other patients who have known vascular disease, e.g. previous myocardial infarction.
- All people with diabetes should be screened on diagnosis, when optimal control is achieved, and if control ever deteriorates or insulin is started. Fasting levels are the most reliable, if possible (this may be difficult to arrange in people with type 1 diabetes).
- Fibrates may be preferable because they also benefit the clotting system and possibly diabetic control. However, statins are often the first choice in view of the 4S trial and other evidence.
- Action levels: recent trials suggest that a cholesterol level of >5.5 mmol/l should be treated for secondary prevention in people with cardiovascular disease.
- Recent evidence does, however, suggest that levels of low-density lipoproteins (LDL) are important in assessing vascular risk and treatment to lower these could be considered. The percentage reduction in LDL levels is possibly more important than the actual level achieved.

female patients with diabetes was 60% in men and 100% in women respectively, compared with values for non-diabetic individuals. The box above gives suggestions about screening for cholesterol in people with diabetes.

Epidemiological studies have demonstrated that even mild impairment of glucose tolerance is associated with an increase in atherosclerosis. This may imply that hyperglycaemia is an important factor, although it is possible that other factors, as yet unidentified, are involved. Hypertension is approximately twice as common in patients with diabetes as in age-matched people without diabetes. It is more frequent in type 1 diabetes than in type 2 diabetes. Obesity and the presence of renal disease are associated with hypertension in diabetes; however, it has been shown that these links extend further. Epidemiologically, there is an association between blood glucose levels (after a standard load) and both systolic and diastolic blood pressure, independent of body weight. The United Kingdom Prospective Study (UKPDS) demonstrated that the morbidity and mortality associated with cardiovascular complications in people with type 2 diabetes can be reduced by the identification of risk factors and tighter control of weight, blood pressure and hyperlipidaemia.

The *National Service Framework for Coronary Heart Disease: Modern Standards and Service Models* includes the following recommendations as one of its 12 standards:

- preventing CHD in high-risk patients in primary care: GPs and primary health care teams should identify all people at significant risk of cardiovascular disease but who have not yet developed symptoms, and offer them appropriate advice and treatment to reduce their risk

Treating myocardial infarction patients with insulin has been shown to improve prognosis, particularly in those not already receiving insulin (see the DIGAMI – Diabetes Mellitus Insulin Glucose Infusion in Acute Myocardial Infarction – study).

SUMMARY

Cardiac disease and diabetes mellitus

- Diabetes increases (by two three times) the risk of cardiac disease – a common cause of morbidity and mortality.
- Hyperglycaemia is an important factor.
- Other important factors are thought to be involved, but not yet identified.
- Hypertension is more frequent in type 1 than in type 2 diabetes.
- Treating patients with diabetes and myocardial infarction with insulin improves prognosis.

Aspirin treatment in diabetes

Diabetes UK is now recommending that people with diabetes in the groups below should be offered aspirin treatment, or should obtain it for themselves. Anyone considering starting aspirin treatment should initially discuss this with a member of the diabetes care team: a doctor, nurse, pharmacist or podiatrist, taking this information with them.

Aspirin treatment should be definitely considered for those who are or have been:

- smokers
- overweight (with a BMI > 25)
- from an Indo-Asian background
- high blood pressure > 140/80 mmHg (with or without treatment), but if untreated < 150/90
- microalbuminuria or albuminuria (protein in the urine)
- diabetic retinopathy
- a family history of coronary heart disease (CHD)
- dyslipidaemia (high cholesterol levels: total; >5.0 mmol/l; LDL ≥ 3.0 mmol/l; HDL ≤ 0.9 mmol/l)

Table 21.1 Targets for metabolic control and the control of cardiovascular risk factors in people with diabetes

	Good	Borderline	Poor
Total cholesterol (mmol/l)	<5.0	5.0–6.5	>6.5
HDL-cholesterol (mmol/l)	>1.1	0.9–1.1	<0.9
Fasting triglycerides (mmol/l)	<1.7	1.7–2.2	>2.2
Body mass index (kg/m^2)			
Males	20–25	26–27	> 27
Females	19–24	25–26	> 26
Blood pressure (mmHg)	< 130/80[a]	140/80[b]–160/95	> 160/95
Smoking status	Non-smoker	Smoker	Smoker

[a] Varies according to different guidelines. Stricter targets are advocated for younger people and for individuals with microvascular or macrovascular complications.
[b] UKPDS recommends that treatment is indicated if > 140/80.
Reproduced with permission from Chambers R, Stead J, Wakley G (2001). *Diabetes Matters in Primary Care*. Oxford: Radcliffe Medical Press.

■ a CHD risk >15% over the next 10 years from the coronary risk prediction
■ other accepted conditions such as angina, previous heart attack, stroke, transient ischaemic attacks, atrial fibrillation and peripheral vascular disease.

Exceptions to this would be those who cannot tolerate aspirin, such as those with known peptic ulceration or those who fall into an unusually low-risk group, e.g.:

■ aspirin allergy
■ bleeding tendency
■ anticoagulation therapy
■ past history of gastrointestinal bleeding
■ concurrent use of drugs to prevent gastrointestinal bleeding
■ active hepatic disease
■ history of aspirin-induced asthma.

The more risk factors, the more likely that aspirin treatment will be beneficial. The dosage recommended is at least 75 mg aspirin daily.

21

Further reading

Alexander WD (1998). *Diabetic Retinopathy: A guide for diabetic care teams.* Oxford: Blackwell Science.

Anderson AR, Christiansen IS, Anderson AK et al. (1983). Diabetic nephropathy in type I (insulin-dependent) diabetes, an epidemiological study. *Diabetologia* **25**: 496–501.

Caird FI, Pirie A, Ramsell TG (1969). In: *Diabetes and the Eye.* Oxford: Blackwell Scientific Publications.

Carroll R (1992). Kidney damage in diabetes. *Nursing* **5**(6): 17–20.

Chambers R, Stead J, Wakley G (2001). *Diabetes Matters in Primary Care.* Oxford: Radcliffe Medical Press.

Deckert T, Pulsen IE, Larsen M (1978). Prognosis of diabetes with diabetes before the age of 31. *Diabetologia* **14**: 363–70.

Department of Health (2000). *National Service Framework for Coronary Heart Disease.* London: Department of Health.

Department of Health (2001). *National Service Framework for Coronary Heart Disease: Modern Standards and Service Models.* London: Department of Health.

Diabetes UK (2000) *Advisory Panel Final Report to the UK National Screening Committee.* London: Diabetes UK. (Website: www.diabetic-retinopathy.screening.nhs.uk/recommendations.html)

Diabetic Retinopathy Study Research Group (1981). Photocoagulation treatment of proliferative diabetic retinopathy: clinical application of diabetic retinopathy study (DRS) findings. DRS Report No 8. *Ophthalmology* **88**: 583–600.

Edmonds ME (1985). The neuropathic ulcer. *Practical Diabetes* **2**(1): 46–7.

Elkeles RS, Wolfe IHN (1991). The diabetic foot. *British Medical Journal* **303**: 1053–5.

Geiss LS, Herman WH, Teutsch SM (1985). Diabetes and renal mortality in the United States. *American Journal of Public Health* **75**: B25–6.

Hale PI (1984). Why do diabetic patients suffer from coronary artery disease? *Practical Diabetes* **1**(2): 22–35.

Hansson L et al. (1998). The Hypertension Optimal Treatment (HOT) Study: 24 month data on blood pressure and tolerability. *Lancet* 1998; **351**: 1755–612.

HMSO (1988). *Causes of blindness and partial sight amongst adults.* London: HMSO.

Joint Working Party on Diabetic Renal Failure of the British Diabetic Association, The Renal Association and The Research Unit of The Royal College of Physicians (1988). Renal failure in the UK: deficient provision of care in 1985. *Diabetic Medicine* **5**:79–84.

Kannel WB, McGee DC (1979). Diabetes and cardiovascular disease: The Framingham Study. *Journal of the American Medical Association* **241**: 2035.

Klein BE, Klein R, Moss SE (1985). Prevalence of cataracts in a population based study of persons with diabetes mellitus. *Ophthalmology* **92**: 1191–6.

Kohner EM (1978). The evolution and natural history of diabetic retinopathy. *International Ophthalmology Clinics* **18**: 1–16.

McCulloch DK, Young RJ, Prescott IW et al. (1984). The natural history of impotence in diabetic men. *Diabetologia* **26**: 437–40.

Malmberg K for the DIGAMI Study Group (1997). Prospective randomised study of intensive insulin treatment on long term survival after acute myocardial infarction in patients with diabetes mellitus. *British Medical Journal* **314**: 1512–15.

Mogensen CE (1984). Microalbuminuria predicts clinical proteinuria and early mortality in maturity onset diabetes. *New England Journal of Medicine* **310**: 356–60.

Murphy RP, Nanda M, Plotnick L, Enger C, Vitale S, Patz A (1990). The relationship of puberty to diabetic retinopathy. *Archives of Ophthalmology* **108**: 215–18.

Ryder REJ, Dent MT, Ward ID (1992). Testing for diabetic neuropathy, part two, autonomic neuropathy. *Practical Diabetes* **9**(2): 56–60.

Stamler J, Rhomberg P, Schoenberger IA et al. (1975). Multi-variate analysis of the relationship of seven variables to blood pressure. Findings of the Chicago Heart Association Detection Project in Industry 1962–1972. *Journal of Chronic Disease* **28**: 527–48.

UKPDS 33. *Lancet* 1998; **352**: 837–53.

UKPDS 34. *Lancet* 1998; **352**: 854–65.

UKPDS 35. *BMJ* 2000; **321**: 405–12.

UKPDS 36. *BMJ* 2000; **321**: 412–19.

UKPDS 38. *BMJ* 1998; **317**: 703–13.

UKPDS 39. *BMJ* 1998; **317**: 713–20.

Watkins PI (1988). *ABC of Diabetes.* London: BMJ Publishing Group.

Watkins PJ, Drury PL, Howell SL (1996). *Diabetes and its Management,* 5th edn. Oxford: Blackwell Science.

Williams JG (1991). Diabetic autonomic neuropathy. *Practical Diabetes* **2**(2): 4–5.

Wood D, Durrington P, Poulter N, McInnes G, Rees A, Wray R (1998). Joint recommendations on prevention of coronary heart disease in clinical practice. *Heart* **80**(suppl 2): S1–S29.

Working Group on Hypertension and Diabetes (1987). Statements on hypertension and diabetes: final report. *Archives of Internal Medicine* **147**: 830–42.

21

New insights

There is continuing new evidence and insight into the management of type 2 diabetes. Six recent relevant studies or pieces of research are summarised below.

United Kingdom Prospective Diabetes Study (UKPDS)

Key points

- The largest clinical study of diabetes ever conducted.
- It studied the effect of intensive treatment of type 2 diabetes in reducing long-term complications.
- It demonstrated that long-term complications are reduced with intensive therapy.
- It found that a reduction in HbA1c of 1% was associated with 14% fewer myocardial infarctions, 21% fewer deaths related to diabetes and 37% fewer microvascular complications.
- It demonstrated that type 2 diabetes is a serious and progressive disease and never 'mild'.
- It found that up to 50% of people with type 2 diabetes have long-term complications on diagnosis, emphasising the need for early detection and screening of those in high-risk groups.
- The key treatment targets, reducing long-term complications in the study, relate to tight blood pressure and intensive blood glucose control.
- Two papers (35 and 36) show the close relationship between complications and control of bood glucose and blood pressure.

Prevalence and incidence of type 2 diabetes in the UK (Poole 1998)

- It is estimated that over 1 million people are currently diagnosed with type 2 diabetes in the UK.
- Another million may be undiagnosed.

- Over 100,000 people are diagnosed with diabetes each year in the UK (one person every 5 minutes).
- The number of cases among men is significantly higher than among women.
- This is a marked change from the position in the 1950s and 1960s, when cases among women were higher.
- The cause of this shift is unknown.
- Advancing age of the population, obesity and a sedentary lifestyle are thought to be contributing factors to increasing numbers of cases.
- Groups at particularly high risk are those aged over 40 years who are overweight or of Asian or African–Caribbean origin, or have a family history of diabetes or a prior history of gestational diabetes.

Primary Care Diabetes – a national survey

A national survey in England and Wales (Pierce et al., 2000) aimed to describe the following:

- The extent and organisation of general practice diabetes care.
- Primary care perceptions of support by secondary care.
- Cooperation with secondary care.
- Educational experience in diabetes of doctors and nurses in primary care.

The enquiry confirmed that, over the past decade, the focus of diabetes care has shifted and most is provided in general practice. There are significant geographical variations in the delivery of primary diabetes care.

One in five practices in England and Wales was surveyed. The response to the survey was 70%.

Some results

- Median number of diabetes patients per practice is 110.
- Of patients, 75% with diabetes are described as having most or all of their diabetes care in general practice.
- Of practices, 68% had a special interest in diabetes.
- Of practices, 96% had diabetes registers.
- Of practices, 87% used their registers for call and recall.
- Of practices, 77% had fully computerised registers.

Key messages

- A large volume of diabetes care takes place in primary care.
- Those providing it are very enthusiastic.
- Nurses are important and the key to success.

The Hypertension Optimal Treatment (HOT) Study

- A very large study (18,790 patients) to investigate the optimum target diastolic blood pressure.
- A subgroup of these hypertensive patients also had diabetes (1,501 patients).
- In patients with diabetes, a diastolic blood pressure of 80 mmHg led to a reduction of severe cardiovascular events by 51%, compared with a diastolic blood pressure of 90 mmHg.
- The reduction in morbidity was accompanied by a parallel improvement in well-being.
- UKPDS data (paper 36) show that patients with a normal systolic blood pressure (130 mmHg) have a lower risk of coronary heart disease.
- Thus, the target blood pressure for people with diabetes is 130/80.

Islet cell transplants

- Where insulin-secreting pancreatic β cells have failed completely, transplanting functioning islet cells from a donor is currently the only hope for restoring insulin secretion.
- The technique has been tried in the past but usually fails as a result of allograft rejection.
- However, recent trials (conducted in Canada) resulted in 13 of 15 patients being free of insulin injections a year or more after islet cell transplantation, while being treated with a triple immunosuppressant cocktail.
- Islet cell transplantation trials using donor pancreases are now planned for seven centres in the UK, once legal, ethical, funding and practical issues have been resolved.

The DECODE Study Group

Glucose tolerance and mortality: comparison of WHO and American Diabetic Association diagnostic criteria

- The ADA proposed that diabetes be defined by a fasting plasma glucose of 7.0 mmol/l alone and did not recommend the use of the oral glucose tolerance test.
- WHO recommended the oral glucose tolerance test should be used only if the blood glucose concentration is in the uncertain range 5.5–11.1 mmol/l.

For the diagnosis of diabetes mellitus, WHO recommend the same fasting concentration as the ADA, *as well* as a 2-h glucose concentration of at least 11.1 mmol/l.

- A high degree of disagreement in the fasting and 2-h classifications has been seen between the two recommendations in European populations.
- DECODE assessed mortality associated with the ADA fasting glucose criteria compared with the WHO 2-h post-challenge glucose criteria.
- Data from 13 prospective European cohort studies was examined, including 18,048 men and 7,316 women aged 30 years or older. Mean follow-up was 7.3 years.

Key findings

- Compared with people who had normal fasting glucose (< 6.1 mmol/l), people with newly diagnosed diabetes by the ADA fasting criteria (> 7.0 mmol/l) had hazard ratios for death of 1.81 (men) and 1.79 (women).
- For impaired fasting glucose (6.1–6.9 mmol/l) the hazard ratios were 1.21 and 1.08.
- For the WHO criteria (> 11.1 mmol/l) the ratios for newly diagnosed diabetes were 2.02 in men and 2.77 in women.
- For impaired fasting glucose (7.8–11.1 mmol/l) the ratios were 1.51 and 1.60.
- Within each fasting-glucose classification, mortality increased with increasing 2-h glucose.
- For 2-h glucose classifications of impaired glucose tolerance and diabetes, there was no trend for increasing fasting glucose concentrations.

Significance

- An increase in 2-h glucose resulted in a significant increase in mortality, independent of fasting glucose.
- Fasting blood glucose is not as satisfactory as 2-h blood glucose for the prediction of mortality.

Further reading

Budd S et al. (1998). Poole Study. *Diabetic Medicine* (suppl 2): 511.

DECODE Study (1999). DECODE Study Group. *Lancet* **354**: 617–21.

Hansson L et al. (1998). The Hypertension Optimal Treatment (HOT) Study: 24 month data on blood pressure and tolerability. *Lancet* 1998; **351**: 1755–612.

Pierce M, Agarwal G, Ridout D. A survey of diabetes care in general practice in England and Wales, *British Journal of General Practice* 2000; 50: 542–45.

UKPDS 33. *Lancet* 1998; **352**: 837–53.

UKPDS 34. *Lancet* 1998; **352**: 854–65.

UKPDS 35. *BMJ* 2000; **321**: 405–12.

UKPDS 36. *BMJ* 2000; **321**: 412–19.

UKPDS 38. *BMJ* 1998; **317**: 703–13.

UKPDS 39. *BMJ* 1998; **317**: 713–20

22

Appendices

Appendix I

The St Vincent Declaration: Diabetes Care and Research in Europe

Representatives of government health departments and patients' organisations from all European countries met with diabetes experts under the aegis of the Regional Office of the World Health Organization (WHO) and the International Diabetes Federation (IDF) in St Vincent, Italy on 10–12 October 1989. They unanimously agreed upon the following recommendations and urged that they should be presented in all countries throughout Europe for implementation:

Diabetes mellitus is a major and growing European health problem, a problem at all ages and in all countries. It causes prolonged ill-health and early death. It threatens at least ten million European citizens.

It is within the power of national Government and Health Departments to create conditions in which a major reduction in this heavy burden of disease and death can be achieved. Countries should give formal recognitions to the diabetes problem and deploy resources for its solution. Plans for the prevention, identification and treatment of diabetes, and particularly its complications – blindness, renal failure, gangrene and amputation, aggravated coronary heart disease and stroke – should be formulated at local, national and European regional levels. Investment now will earn great dividends in reduction of human misery and in massive savings of human and material resources.

General goals and five-year targets listed below can be achieved by the organised activities of the medical services in active partnership with diabetic citizens, their families, friends and workmates and their organisations; in the management of their own diabetes and the education for it; in national, regional and international organisations for disseminating information about health maintenance; in promoting and applying research.

General goals for people – children and adults – with diabetes

- Sustained improvement in health experience and a life approaching normal expectation in quality and quantity.
- Prevention and cure of diabetes and of its complications by intensifying research effort.

Five-year targets

Elaborate, initiate and evaluate comprehensive programmes for detection and control of diabetes and of its complications with self-care and community support as major components.

Raise awareness in the population and among health care professionals of the present opportunities and the future needs for prevention of the complications of diabetes itself.

Organise training and teaching in diabetes management and care for people of all ages with diabetes, for their families, friends and working associates and for the health care team.

Ensure that care for children with diabetes is provided by individuals and teams specialised in the management both of diabetes and of children, and that families with a diabetic child get the necessary social, economic and emotional support.

Reinforce existing centres of excellence in diabetes care, education and research. Create new centres where the need and potential exist.

Promote independence, equity and self-sufficiency for all people with diabetes – children, adolescents, those in the working years of life and the elderly.

Remove hindrances to the fullest possible integration of the diabetic citizen into society.

Implement effective measures for the prevention of costly complications:

- Reduce new blindness due to diabetes by one-third or more.
- Reduce numbers of people entering end-stage diabetic renal failure by at least one-third.
- Reduce by one-half the rate of limb amputation for diabetic gangrene.
- Cut morbidity and mortality from coronary heart disease in the diabetic by vigorous programmes of risk factor reduction.
- Achieve pregnancy outcome in the woman with diabetes that approximates that of the non-diabetic woman.

Establish monitoring and control systems using state of the art information technology for quality assurance of diabetes health care provision and for laboratory and technical procedures in diabetes diagnosis, treatment and self-management.

Promote European and international collaboration in programmes of diabetes research and development through national, regional and WHO agencies and in active partnership with diabetes patients' organisations.

Take urgent action in the spirit of the WHO programme, 'Health for Life' to establish joint machinery between WHO and IDF, European Region, to initiate, accelerate and facilitate the implementation of these recommendations.

At the conclusion of the St Vincent meeting, all those attending formally pledged themselves to strong and decisive action in seeking implementations of the recommendations on their return home.

Appendix II

St Vincent Declaration recommendations for the care of children

These are the St Vincent Declaration recommendations for the care of children and adolescents with diabetes.

Diagnosis

Early symptoms of diabetes in children and adolescents (such as thirst, increased urine production and weight loss) should be made familiar not only to all health care professionals but also to the general population. Information about diabetes should be spread through the mass media and included in school curricula. Test materials for the measurement of glucose in urine should be available to all health care professionals.

Treatment

Newly diagnosed patients should be treated at units whose staff have specialised knowledge of diabetes in children and adolescents. The diabetes care team should include a paediatric diabetologist, a dietitian, a specialist diabetes nurse and a social worker or psychologist.

Long term care should be managed by a paediatrician experienced in the care of diabetic children. The interval between follow up visits should be one to three months, but shorter when needed: for example after major treatment adjustments. Long term glucose control should be estimated by measurement of glycated haemoglobin at least every three months. Growth and pubertal development should be followed regularly and values plotted on growth charts. The general practitioner can handle some acute problems and under exceptional circumstances intermediate consultation but always in consultation with the responsible diabetologist.

Recommendations

Recommendations are made for a standard of care for children and adolescents. They include: education appropriate to age and including the family, school or college. This education should be provided orally and in writing and should encompass information about weekends, holidays and camps.

Recommendations for specialist teams also include:

- Psychological/social support
- Insulin treatment
- Nutrition
- Self-management
- Blood glucose control – targets
- Late vascular complications
- Social rights.

Information

Your guide to better diabetes care: right and roles

This is produced under the auspices of the St Vincent Declaration Steering Committee of IDF/WHO Europe and the Council of the European Region of the IDF.

Further reading

Krans HMJ, Porta M, Keen H, eds (1992). *Diabetes Care and Research in Europe. The St Vincent Declaration action programme. Implementation document.* World Health Organization, Regional Office for Europe, Copenhagen.

Appendix III

What care people with diabetes should expect (information for patients)

The St Vincent Declaration implementation document provides a guideline for people with diabetes. This guideline is reflected in the Diabetes UK leaflet *What Diabetes Care to Expect*, available FREE on request from Diabetes UK. Extracts are reproduced below. Note that this leaflet is for people with diabetes – the 'you' addressed.

Your statutory rights

The following list explains your rights according to the law. If you feel any of these have been broken, it is possible to take your complaint to court.

- You have a right to receive most health care free of charge.
- You have a right to choose the GP you want; but the GP has a right not to accept you, and does not need to give you an explanation. If you are having problems finding a GP you have a right to ask your local health authority to help. You may change your GP whenever you wish and do not need to give advance notice.
- You have a right to see your medical notes (records). However, the holder of the records may refuse to let you see them if he or she thinks it might be harmful to your physical or mental health. They may refuse to let you see any part of your records where a third party is mentioned who does not want you to see that part of the records.
- You have a right to refuse treatment if you do not agree with it, unless the treatment is under the provisions of the Mental Health Act 1983.
- You have a right to have information about you kept confidential by the NHS – it will normally only be used by health professionals in the course of your treatment.
- You have a right to make any reasonable complaint against the NHS. Your complaint will be investigated under the NHS complaints procedure.
- You may have a right to full or part refund of charges for travel costs to hospital, NHS prescriptions, NHS dental treatment, NHS sight tests, glasses and contact lenses, and for NHS wigs and fabric supports. For further information, contact your local Benefits Agency.

What you should expect from the National Health Service (NHS)

You should receive all health services without discrimination because of age, lifestyle, sex, ethnicity, class, religion, disability, sexuality or your ability to pay. The NHS should:

■ treat you with respect and dignity
■ tell you how to contact your diabetes care team
■ treat you with skill and care, and regularly review your clinical needs
■ answer any questions about the quality of the services you are getting
■ provide an interpreting service if English is not your first language, or if you have a sensory impairment or learning difficulties
■ provide information about local health services and how to contact them
■ keep you up to date about your diabetes, its care and treatment (and give you access to a second opinion subject to the agreement of your own GP or consultant).

What care you should expect from your diabetes care team

To achieve the best possible diabetes care, you need to work together with health care professionals as equal members of your diabetes care team. It is essential that you understand your diabetes as well as possible so that you are an effective member of this team.

You need to discuss with your consultant or GP the roles and responsibilities of those providing your diabetes care and to identify the key members of your own diabetes care team.

Members in your diabetes care team

■ Yourself
■ Consultant physician/diabetologist
■ GP
■ Diabetes specialist nurse (DSN)
■ Practice nurse
■ Dietitian
■ Optometrist/ophthalmologist
■ Podiatrist/chiropodist
■ Psychologist
■ Medical specialists
■ Pharmacist.

You may see some members of your diabetes care team more often than others.

When you have just been diagnosed, your diabetes care team should:
- give you a full medical examination
- work with you to make a programme of care which suits you and includes diabetes management goals (see the annual review checklist on pages 80–3)
- arrange for you to talk with a diabetes specialist nurse (or practice nurse) who will explain what diabetes is and discuss your individual treatment and the equipment you will need to use
- arrange for you to talk with a state-registered dietitian, who will want to know what you usually eat, and will give you advice on how to fit your usual diet in with your diabetes. A follow-up meeting should be arranged for more detailed advice
- tell you about your diabetes and the beneficial effects of a healthy diet, exercise and good diabetes control
- discuss the effects of diabetes on your job, driving, insurance, prescription charges and, if you are a driver, whether you need to inform the DVLA and your insurance company
- provide you with regular and appropriate information and education, on food and footcare, for example
- give you information about Diabetes UK services and details of your local Diabetes UK voluntary group.

Once your diabetes is reasonably controlled, you should:
- have access to your diabetes care team at least once a year; in this session, take the opportunity to discuss how your diabetes affects you as well as your diabetes control
- be able to contact any member of your diabetes care team for specialist advice, in person or by phone
- have further education sessions when you are ready for them
- have a formal medical annual review (see pages 80–3) once a year with a doctor experienced in diabetes.

On a regular basis, your diabetes care team should:
- provide continuity of care, ideally from the same doctors and nurses. If this is not possible, the doctors or nurses whom you are seeing should be fully aware of your medical history and background
- work with you continually to review your programme of care, including your diabetes management goals (see the annual review check list on pages 80–3)
- let you share in decisions about your treatment or care
- let you manage your own diabetes in hospital after discussion with your doctor, if you are well enough to do so and that is what you wish
- organise pre- and post-pregnancy advice, together with an obstetric hospital team, if you are planning to become or already are pregnant

- encourage a carer to visit with you, to keep them up to date on diabetes in order to be able to make informed judgements about diabetes care
- encourage the support of friends, partners and/or relatives
- provide you with educational sessions and appointments if you wish
- give you advice on the effects of diabetes and its treatments when you are ill or taking other medication.

Plus

If you are treated by insulin injections you should:
- have frequent visits showing you how to inject, look after your insulin and syringes and dispose of sharps (needles). Also how to test your blood glucose and test for ketones and what the results mean
- be given supplies of, or a prescription for the medication and equipment you need*
- discuss hypoglycaemia (hypos): when and why they may happen and how to deal with them.

If you are treated by tablets you should:
- be given instruction on blood or urine testing and have explained what the results mean
- be given supplies of, or a prescription for, the medication and equipment you need*
- discuss hypoglycaemia (hypos): when and why they may happen and how to deal with them.

If you are treated by diet alone you should:
- be given instruction on blood or urine testing and what the results mean
- be given supplies of equipment you may need.

*Your hospital team will only give you your first prescription. Further prescriptions for medication, test strips, etc. will be provided through your GP.

People with type 1 diabetes and tablet-controlled type 2 diabetes are entitled to free prescriptions for medication. Equipment such as blood glucose meters and finger-pricking devices normally have to be purchased, but test strips, lancets and pen needles are available on prescription. Discuss this with your GP.

A prescription exemption certificate is available from your local health authority or equivalent in Scotland and Northern Ireland.

Your responsibilities

Effective diabetes care is normally achieved by team work, between you and your diabetes care team. Looking after your diabetes and changing your lifestyle to fit in with the demands of diabetes is hard work, but you're worth it!

You will not always get your care right; none of us does, but your diabetes care team is there to support you. Ask questions and request more information especially if you are uncertain or worried about your diabetes and/or treatment. Remember the most important person in the team is you.

The following list of responsibilities is given to help you play your part in your own diabetes care. It is your responsibility:

- to take as much control of your diabetes on a day-to-day basis as you can. The more you know about your own diabetes, the easier this will become
- to learn about and practise self-care which should include dietary education, exercise and monitoring blood glucose levels
- to examine your feet regularly or have someone check them
- to know how to manage your diabetes and when to ask for help if you are ill, e.g. chest infection, flu, or diarrhoea and vomiting
- to know when, where and how to contact your diabetes care team
- to build the diabetes advice discussed with you into your daily life
- to talk regularly with your diabetes care team and ask questions
- to make a list of points to raise at appointments, if you find it helpful
- to attend your scheduled appointments and inform the diabetes care team if you are unable to do so.

Appendix IV

Primary Care Diabetes UK

History

Primary Care Diabetes UK (PCDUK) was launched in November 1996. The launch, supported by the BDA, now Diabetes UK, and the Diabetes Industry Group, took place at an inaugural conference held in London. Conference participants approved the Constitution and elected their first committee. The Chairman (Dr Colin Kenny, General Practitioner, Co. Down) and officers were appointed. The aim of PCDUK was agreed as follows:

> To encourage high quality and culturally sensitive care for people with diabetes within primary care.

Strategic objectives

- To promote awareness and interest in diabetes within primary care.
- To encourage evidence-based practice in diabetes care by the primary care team.
- To promote research and development into the provision of good diabetes care in primary care.
- To promote the interests of people with diabetes, especially those with particular needs.
- To acts as a resource for information about diabetes for the primary care team.
- To promote the integration of diabetes care among health care professionals.
- To contribute actively to discussions on diabetes at a national level.
- To promote appropriate information technology systems and data sets for the management of diabetes.
- To embrace the ideals of the St Vincent Declaration Primary Care Group Europe of which Primary Care Diabetes UK is a division.

PCDUK – a professional section of Diabetes UK

■ PCDUK is a professional section of Diabetes UK, existing alongside the Secondary Care, Basic and Clinical Science and Education sections.

■ It is a coordinating group whose membership includes representation from all Diabetes UK professional sections, and links them together to promote integration in diabetes care.

■ The Chairs of each section, while in post, are automatically invited to join the Diabetes UK Board of Trustees.

■ It is a division of the St Vincent Declaration Primary Care Group Europe, with a designated committee member who has liaison responsibilities.

What Diabetes UK offers PCDUK members

■ PCDUK website: www.diabetes.org

■ Opportunities to keep up to date with research news and innovations in diabetes care.

■ Professional development and continuing education through a range of Diabetes UK conferences, meetings and events (at preferential rates).

■ Support and representation through Diabetes UK links with the Department of Health and National Professional bodies, associations and agencies.

■ Links with other health care professionals, fostering an integrated, multidisciplinary approach to diabetes health care.

■ Access to all Diabetes UK services and resources – including research information, reports, leaflets, books, videos and disks on all aspects of diabetes and diabetes health care.

■ Careline – information and support for people with diabetes and professionals.

What membership of PCDUK means

To provide a new national standard of diabetes care in the UK that meets the needs and expectations of people with diabetes and is realistically achievable and within available resources, health care providers increasingly recognise that they need to:

■ work together

- learn together
- acquire new skills
- keep up to date
- share what they know
- value each other.

Membership of PCDUK offers opportunities for people working in primary care to keep up to date and share ideas about providing care.

PCDUK is a forum in which working relationships and integrated diabetes care can flourish in association with other Diabetes UK professional sections.

Most importantly, people with diabetes and those close to them will know that PCDUK members are interested in diabetes, committed to providing high-quality, evidence-based health care, and belong to a national network dedicated to the delivery of 'culturally sensitive' diabetes care.

Joining PCDUK

Membership of PCDUK is open to all professionals in the primary and community setting interested and involved in providing health care for people with diabetes and their families. Full details of membership eligibility and committee structure, as laid down in the Constitution, are available from the committee secretaries, Diabetes UK. Please address all enquiries to:

Primary Care Diabetes UK
Diabetes UK
10 Queen Anne Street
London W1G 9LH
Tel: 020 7323 1531
Fax: 020 7637 3644

Appendix V

Diabetes Industry Group

The Diabetes Industry Group (DIG) was instrumental in the launch of PCDUK. At the end of 1998, the DIG decided to expand its remit to all areas of diabetes care.

The DIG has already established goodwill in all areas involved in diabetes and related disorders and remains committed to supporting secondary care.

It is the firm conviction of the current members of the DIG that more members from industry would greatly strengthen its activities and influence within the NHS.

Current members of the DIG

- Abbott Laboratories MediSense Products
- Aventis Pharma Ltd
- Bayer plc
- Becton Dickinson UK
- Eli Lilly and Company
- GlaxoSmithKline
- Lifescan
- Merck Sharp & Dohme
- Novartis Pharmaceuticals UK Ltd
- Novo Nordisk
- Pfizer Ltd
- Roche Diagnostics Ltd
- Servier Laboratories
- Takeda UK Ltd

Objectives

- To foster a positive image of the health care industry
- To act together as a voice of the industry in the field of diabetes and related disorders
- To assist in raising the profile of diabetes and related disorders
- To help in achieving the targets of the St Vincent Declaration
- To enhance diabetes education.

Appendix VI

Requirements of Health Authorities

The outline arrangements for diabetes in general practice are as follows.

Aims, responsibilities and educational needs relating to existing and new arrangements

New arrangements for banded/costed health promotion clinics reflect objectives set out in the 'Health of the Nation'. Initially, they will focus on three main areas – smoking cessation, coronary heart disease and stroke. Health Authorities expect general practitioners to run disease management programmes for asthma and diabetes, each attracting an annual allowance for general practitioners involved in the schemes.

Practices must set up an organised programme for the care of patients with diabetes mellitus.

What practices have to do

- Keep an up-to-date register of all patients with diabetes.
- Ensure that a systematic call and recall of patients on this register is taking place either to hospital or to the practice.
- Provide education for newly diagnosed diabetics, ensuring that all newly diagnosed patients and/or their carers receive appropriate education and advice on the management and prevention of secondary complications of their diabetes.
- Ensure that all patients with diabetes or their carers receive continuing education.
- Ensure that, at initial diagnosis and at least annually, a full review of the patient's health is carried out including checks for potential complications and a review of the patient's own monitoring records.
- Prepare an individual management plan with the patient.
- Work together with other professionals such as dietitians and chiropodists (podiatrists) and ensure that they are appropriately trained in the management of diabetes.
- Refer patients to secondary care where appropriate and to relevant support agencies.

- Maintain adequate records of performance and results of these procedures, including information from other people involved in the care of patients.
- Audit the care of patients with diabetes against the above criteria.

Reference

NHS Management Executive. 12/01/93. *GP contract health promotion package: guidance on implementation.*

Appendix VII

British Diabetic Association recommendations for the management of diabetes in primary care

Aims

The overall aim of any system of diabetes care is:

To enable people with diabetes to achieve a quality of life and life expectancy similar to that of the general population by reducing the complications of diabetes.

Good metabolic control and management of cardiovascular risk factors are key to the achievement of this aim. The maintenance of near normal blood glucose levels is crucial to the prevention of the microvascular complications of diabetes – blindness, diabetic renal disease and diabetic neuropathy – as well as the achievement of symptom control and the avoidance of the acute metabolic crises of hypoglycaemia and ketoacidosis. Attention to cardiovascular risk factors, including smoking, hyperlipidaemia, hypertension, obesity and a lack of physical activity, is equally important. Regular monitoring and appropriate management of blood glucose control and cardiovascular risk factors are therefore essential.

The active involvement of patients in their own care is crucial for good diabetes management – it is the person with diabetes who plays the most important role in this process, and hence his or her motivation is essential. Effective, ongoing education, matched to each patient's ability and capacity to learn, can enable the person with diabetes to take responsibility for his or her own health. People with diabetes should also be empowered to obtain maximum benefit from health care services so that, as far as possible, they are able to participate in activities open to those without diabetes.

The early detection and treatment of many established complications can reduce morbidity and health care costs. In retinopathy, for example, the detection of early retinal disease followed by laser treatment can prevent blindness. Planned follow-up with effective surveillance for complications is therefore essential.

The following targets have been agreed in the St Vincent Declaration:

- Reduce cases of blindness by at least one-third.
- Reduce numbers of people entering end-stage renal failure by at least one-third.
- Reduce rate of limb amputation for diabetic gangrene by at least half.
- Cut mortality and morbidity from coronary heart disease in people with diabetes.
- Improve the outcome of diabetic pregnancies.

Objectives

The main objectives of diabetes care are therefore to ensure:

- The provision of appropriate education to equip people with diabetes with the knowledge, skills and motivation to manage their diabetes care, and to modify their lifestyle in such a way as to maximise their well-being.
- The maintenance of blood glucose control at as near physiological levels as possible, while at the same time aiming to achieve as near normal a lifestyle as possible, through regular monitoring of metabolic control and appropriate management, thereby minimising the likelihood of people with diabetes developing short-term and long-term complications.
- The identification and appropriate management of individuals with cardiovascular risk factors, including:
  - ◆ smoking
  - ◆ hyperlipidaemia
  - ◆ hypertension
  - ◆ obesity
  - ◆ lack of physical activity.
- The early identification and appropriate management of individuals with long-term complications of diabetes, in order to reduce:
  - ◆ ischaemic heart disease: angina, myocardial infarction and cardiac failure
  - ◆ foot ulceration and limb amputation caused by peripheral vascular disease and diabetic nerve damage
  - ◆ blindness and visual impairment resulting from diabetic eye disease
  - ◆ stroke and other cerebrovascular disease
  - ◆ end-stage renal failure caused by diabetic renal disease.
- The strict maintenance of blood glucose control before conception and throughout pregnancy in diabetic women in order to reduce fetal loss during pregnancy, stillbirths and congenital malformations, and neonatal problems in their offspring.

Provision of diabetes care within primary care

The British Diabetic Association (BDA) produced a leaflet for people with diabetes entitled *Diabetes Care – what you should expect.* The leaflet, which is available from the BDA, explains what treatment and advice patients should expect from their health care team.

The leaflet stresses the importance of patients understanding their diabetes so that they are enabled to become effective members of the health care team. Increasingly, patients will therefore expect to receive the level of care specified in the leaflet, whether their diabetes care is being provided in a hospital or primary care setting.

Although practice nurses and other members of the primary health care team are providing an increasing proportion of diabetes care, general practitioners (GPs) have overall responsibility for ensuring that all patients with diabetes registered on their lists are involved in a planned programme of diabetes care, tailored to meet the needs of each individual patient.

The first step to achieving this aim is to identify all patients registered with the GP who have clinically diagnosed diabetes. This will involve the setting up and maintenance of a practice register of patients with diabetes, which should ideally be computerised. Patients ascertained in this way can then be categorised according to whether or not they are involved in a planned programme of care and, if so, where this care is being provided. Mechanisms should be in place for collating practice-held data to enable the district-wide audit and planning of diabetes services.

The care of patients with diabetes is always a collaborative effort involving a number of different health professionals. The appropriate setting for the various elements of a programme of diabetes care will vary according to the needs of the particular patient. It will be for the members of the primary health care team, in collaboration with members of the specialist diabetes team, to negotiate and agree where each element of care should take place. GPs should provide planned follow-up for any patient not being followed up elsewhere.

A clear management plan should be developed with each individual patient so that the responsibility for the various aspects of care is clear. The components of the management should be discussed and agreed with each patient. Communication between the different disciplines is the key to successful care. A patient-held record can help to facilitate the process (see Appendix IX); other approaches are also being developed, including the facility to print out copies of the computerised record held by the health professionals involved and the development of electronic unified medical records and smart cards.

> **Key elements of effective diabetes care**
>
> - A planned programme of care for all patients with diabetes.
> - Clear management plans agreed with each patient, tailored to meet the needs of individuals and their carers.
> - Practice-based diabetes register to facilitate regular call and recall of patients.

A planned programme of diabetes care should include systems for ensuring:

- Early identification of patients with diabetes
- Assessment and initial management of the newly diagnosed
- Initial stabilisation, symptom control and education of these patients – including dietary assessment
- Identification and reassessment of those lost to follow-up
- Regular review and maintenance of metabolic control in all patients with diagnosed diabetes
- Regular review and management of cardiovascular risk factors
- On-going education for all patients with diagnosed diabetes
- Management of acute complications
- Detection and management of long-term complications
- Ongoing quality assurance.

Patients within certain agreed groups are better followed up by a specialist diabetes team, including:

- All children and adolescents
- All women considering pregnancy or who are already pregnant
- Any patient whom the GP feels is in need of specialist advice regarding the management of metabolic control, cardiovascular risk factors or diabetic complications.

To meet the needs of all patients with diagnosed diabetes, primary and specialist care should be integrated. The aim should be to ensure that patients are managed in the most appropriate setting.

Ideally, district diabetes policies should be agreed which set out referral criteria for patients with diabetes, including the timing and route of such referrals. Such criteria must also take account of the different levels of skill and interest in the management of diabetes among primary health care teams.

After discussion, it may be decided that some patients, currently being followed up by a specialist team, could in future either be followed up by the primary health care team, or be the subject of integrated/shared care between the primary care and specialist teams.

Reference

British Diabetic Association. Diabetes Advisory Committee (1997). *Recommendations for the Management of Diabetes in Primary Care.* London: BDA (These recommendations are now out of print.)

Appendix VIII

Resources for the provision of diabetes care

A new national education and resource initiative

Warwick Diabetes Care (University of Warwick) was launched in November 2000. It provides coherent point of contact for all those involved in providing diabetes care in the following ways:

- providing and promoting multidisciplinary diabetes education courses for health care professionals
- undertaking and supporting applied diabetes research
- developing practical resources and people networks.

Warwick Diabetes Care
Tel: 024 7657 2958
Fax: 024 7657 3959
Email: diabetes@warwick.ac.uk
Website: www.diabetescare.warwick.ac.uk

Practical, useful and interesting books for people with diabetes

Bilous RW (2000). *Understanding Diabetes*. London: Family Doctor Publications.
Cutting D (2001). *Stop that Heart Attack!*, 2nd edn. London: Class Publishing.
*Day J (1998). *Living with Diabetes: The BDA guide for those treated with insulin*. Chichester: John Wiley & Sons.
*Day J (1998). *Living with Diabetes: The BDA guide for those treated with diet and tablets*. Chichester: John Wiley & Sons.
*Elliott J (1987). *If Your Child is Diabetic*. London: Sheldon Press.
*Estridge B (1996). *Diabetes and Your Teenager*. London: Thorsons.
Hart JT, Fahey T, Savage W (1999). *High Blood Pressure at Your Fingertips*, 2nd edn. London: Class Publishing.
Hillson R (1996). *Diabetes: The complete guide*. London: Vermilion.
Hillson R (1996). *PHG Diabetes beyond 40*, 2nd edn. London: Optima.

Hillson R (1996). *Late Onset Diabetes*. London: Vermilion.

Jackson G (2000). *Heart Health at Your Fingertips*. London: Class Publishing.

Knopfler A (1992). *Diabetes and Pregnancy*. London: Little, Brown & Co.

*Sönsken P, Fox C, Judd S (1998). *Diabetes at your Fingertips*, 4th edn. London: Class Publishing.

Titles marked * are available from Diabetes UK.

Multimedia

Learning Diabetes (insulin treated) and *Learning Diabetes (non-insulin treated)*: multimedia patient education programmes produced as a package called 'Managing Your Health' by Interactive Eurohealth.

For information, please telephone, or fax, 01394 412141 or email sales@interactiveeurohealth.com

Useful books for the primary care team

Alexander WD (1998). *Diabetic Retinopathy: A guide for diabetes care teams*. Oxford: Blackwell Science.

Areffio A, Hill RD, Leigh O (1992). *Diabetes and Primary Eye Care*. Oxford: Blackwell Science.

Campbell IW, Lebovitz H (1996). *Fast Facts – Diabetes Mellitus*. Oxford: Health Press.

Chambers R, Stead J, Wakley G (2001). *Diabetes Matters in Primary Care*. Oxford: Radcliffe Medical Press.

Connor H, Boulton A (1989). *Diabetes in Practice*. Chichester: John Wiley & Sons.

Dornhorst D, Hadden DR (eds) (1996). *Diabetes and Pregnancy. An international approach to diagnosis and management*. Chichester: John Wiley & Sons Ltd.

Edmonds ME, Foster AVM (2000). *Managing the Diabetic Foot*. Oxford: Blackwell Science.

Feher M (1993). *Hypertension in Diabetes Mellitus*. London: Martin Dunitz.

Foster MC, Cole M (1996). *Impotence: A guide to management*. London: Martin Dunitz.

Fox C, MacKinnon M (2001). *Vital Diabetes*, 2nd edn. London: Class Publishing.

Fox C, Pickering A (1995). *Diabetes in the Real World*. London: Class Publishing.

Gatling W, Hill R, Kirby M (1997) *Shared Care for Diabetes*. Oxford: ISIS Medical Media.

Jerreat L (1999). *Diabetes for Nurses*. London: Whurr Publishers.

Pickup J, Williams G (1997). *Textbook of Diabetes*, 2nd edn. Oxford: Blackwell Science.

Shillitoe R (1994). *Counselling People with Diabetes*. Leicester: BPS Books.

Watkins PJ, Drury PL, Howell SL (1996). *Diabetes and Its Management*, 5th edn. Oxford: Blackwell Science.

Williams G, Pickup J (1998). *Handbook of Diabetes*. Oxford: Blackwell Science.

Wise PH (1994). *Knowing about Diabetes for Insulin Dependent Diabetics*, 2nd edn. Foulsham & Co. Ltd.

Useful reports

Alberti KGMM (1999). The diagnosis and classification of diabetes mellitus. *Diabetes Voice* 44: 35–41.

Audit Commission (2000). *Test Times: A review of diabetes services in England and Wales*. London: Audit Commission.

British Diabetic Association/Department of Health (1995). *Report of the St Vincent Task Force for Diabetes*. London: BDA.

British Diabetic Association (1995). *Diabetes in the United Kingdom – 1996. A BDA Report*. London: BDA.

British Diabetic Association (1997). *Recommendations for the Management of Diabetes in Primary Care*. London: BDA.

Hansson L et al. (1998). The Hypertension Optimal Treatment (HOT) Study: 24 month data on blood pressure and tolerability. *Lancet* 1998; **351**: 1755–612.

HMSO (1999). *Saving Lives: Our Healthier Nation*. White Paper, Cm 4386. London: The Stationery Office.

Marks L (1996). *Counting the Cost: The real impact of non-insulin-dependent diabetes*. London: King's Fund/BDA.

Pierce M, Agarwal G, Ridout D (2000). A survey of diabetes care in general practice in England and Wales. *British Journal of General Practice* 2000; **50**: 542–5.

Poole Study (1998). Budd S et al. *Diabetic Medicine* 1998 (suppl 2); 511.

Royal College of Physicians/British Diabetic Association (1993). *Good Practice in the Diagnosis and Treatment of NIDDM*. London: RCP/BDA.

UKPDS 33. *Lancet* 1998; **352**: 837–53.

UKPDS 34. *Lancet* 1998; **352**: 854–65.

UKPDS 35. *BMJ* 2000; **321**: 405–12.

UKPDS 36. *BMJ* 2000; **321**: 412–19.

UKPDS 38. *BMJ* 1998; **317**: 703–13.

UKPDS 39. *BMJ* 1998; **317**: 713–20.

Useful websites

Diabetes UK: www.diabetes.org.uk
Warwick Diabetes Care: www.diabetescare.warwick.ac.uk
British Medical Journal – free access: www.bmj.com
Audit Commission: www.diabetes.audit-commission.gov.uk
Department of Health: www.doh.gov.uk
The NHS Plan: www.nhs.uk/nationalplan
A First Class Service: Quality in the New NHS:
    www.doh.gov.uk/newnhs/quality.htm
Our Healthier Nation: www.doh.gov.uk/ohn.htm
Your Guide to the NHS: www.nhs.uk/nhsguide
National Service Framework for Coronary Heart Disease:
    www.doh.gov.uk/nsf/coronary.htm
International Diabetes Federation: www.idf.org
Medscape – an excellent free resource with a section on diabetes:
    www.medscape.com
Joslin Diabetes Centre – educational website:
    www.joslin.harvard.edu/education

From Diabetes UK

For a comprehensive catalogue of leaflets, books and videos, send for Diabetes UK catalogue and order form to:

Diabetes UK
PO Box 1
Portishead
Bristol BS20 8DJ
Tel: 0800 585088
or 01275 818700

All literature, including the publications listed below, is distributed from the above address and not from 10 Queen Anne Street, London W1M 0BD.
    Diabetes UK also has various resource documents so approach them for a list.

Balance for Beginners

These are a range of magazines for people newly diagnosed with diabetes, or those who would like to update their knowledge.
Diabetes Type 1 (£2.50)
Diabetes for Beginners Type 2 (£2.50)
Just for You (free)
Go for it (£2.50)

Booklets

Diabetes: A guide for African–Caribbean people (£1.80)
Diabetes: A guide for South Asian people (£1.80)
Eating Well with Diabetes (free)

Reports

There are a number of reports produced by Diabetes UK and its professional committees on different aspects of diabetes. These are listed in the catalogue that can be obtained as indicated at start of section.

Posters

There are a number of posters available free for use in clinics.

Videos

There are two videos available (at £11.95): 'Looking after yourself', which is also available in five Asian dialects and 'Diabetes: A guide for African–Caribbean people'.

Journals

Diabetic Medicine
Issued 12 times per year. Can be purchased through professional membership sections of Diabetes UK.

Diabetes Update
Periodic newsletter (free) for the health care professional interested in diabetes; available from Diabetes UK.

Diabetes and Primary Care
Four issues per year. From:
SB Communications Group
15 Manderville Courtyard
142 Battersea Park Road
London SW11 4NB
Tel: 020 7627 1510
Address for subscriptions: FREEPOST LON7814, London SE26 5BR

Journal of Diabetes Nursing
Six issues per year. Subscriptions from SB Communications Group (see above).

Practical Diabetes International
Nine issues per year, available from:
John Wiley & Sons
1 Oldlands Way
Bognor Regis
W. Sussex PO22 9SA
Tel: 012443 779777

Companies

The following provide drugs, equipment, booklets, leaflets, posters, videos, identification cards, monitoring diaries, GP information, training, clinic packs, etc. (local representatives will have specific details of what is available). Please contact the companies at the addresses/telephone numbers given to ascertain exactly what they do provide.

3M Health Care Ltd
3M House Morley Street, Loughborough, Leicestershire LE11 1EP
Tel: 01509 611611
Fax: 01509 237288

Aventis Pharma Ltd
Aventis House, 50 Kings Hill Lane, Kings Hill, West Malling, Kent ME19 4AH
Tel: 01732 584000
Fax: 01732 583080
Website: www.aventis.com

Bayer plc

Diagnostics Division, Bayer House, Strawberry Hill, Newbury, Berks RG14 1JA
Tel: 01635 563000
Fax: 01635 566260
Helpline: 01635 566366
Email: deborahbradbury.db@bayer.co.uk
Website: www.bayer.co.uk

Becton Dickinson UK Ltd

Diabetes Health Care Division, Between Towns Road, Cowley, Oxford OX4 3LY
Tel: 01865 781510
Fax: 01865 781551
Email: bduk_customerservice@europe.bd.com
Website: www.bd.com

BHR

BHR Pharmaceuticals Ltd, 41 Centenary Business Centre, Hammond Close,
Attleborough Fields, Nuneaton, Warwickshire CV11 6RY
Tel: 02476 353742
Fax: 02476 327812

CP Pharmaceuticals

Ash Road North, Wrexham Industrial Estate, Wrexham, Clwyd LL13 9UF
Tel: 01978 661261
Fax: 01978 660130
Email: mail@cppharma.co.uk
Website: www.cppharma.co.uk

GlaxoSmithKline

Stockley Park West, Uxbridge, Middlesex UB11 1BT
Tel: 020 8990 9000
Fax: 020 8990 4321
Helpline: 0800 221 441
Website: www.gsk.com

Golden Key Company (SOS/Talisman)

1 Hare Street, Sheerness, Kent ME12 1AH
Tel: 01795 663403
Fax: 01795 661356
Email: enquiries@goldenkeyuk.com
Website: www.goldenkey.co.uk
For 'diabetic' necklets and bracelets.

Hypoguard UK Ltd
Dock Lane, Melton, Woodridge, Suffolk IP12 1PE
Tel: 01394 387333/4
Fax: 01394 380152
Helpline: 0800 371957
Website: www.hypoguard.com

LifeScan
Division of Ortho Diagnostic Systems Ltd, Enterprise House, Station Road,
Loudwater, High Wycombe, Bucks HP10 9UF
Tel: 01494 450423
Fax: 01494 463299
Helpline: 0800 121200
Website: www.lifescan.com

Lilly Diabetes Care Division
Dextra Court, Chapel Hill, Basingstoke, Hants RG21 5SY
Tel: 01256 315000
Fax: 01256 315058
Email: individuals@lilly.com
Website: www.lilly.com

Medic-Alert Foundation British Isles & Ireland
1 Bridge Wharf, 156 Caledonian Road, London N1 9UU
Tel: 020 7833 3034
Fax: 020 7278 0647
Helpline: 0800 581420
Website: www.medic-alert.co.uk

MediSense Britain Ltd
Mallory House, Vanwell Business Park, Maidenhead, Berks SL6 4UD
Tel: 01628 678900
Fax: 01628 678808
Helpline: 0500 467466
Website: www.abbottlaboratories.com

Merck Pharmaceuticals Ltd
Harrier House, High Street, Yiewsley, West Drayton, Middlesex UB7 7QG
Tel: 01895 452200
Fax: 01895 420605
Email: individuals@merck-lipha.co.uk
Website: www.merck.de

Novartis Pharmaceuticals UK Ltd
Frimley Business Park, Frimley, Camberley, Surrey GU16 7SR
Tel: 01276 692255
Fax: 01276 692508
Medical information line: 01276 692508
Website: www.novartis.com

Novo Nordisk Ltd
Broadfield Park, Brighton Road, Pease Pottage, Crawley, West Sussex RH11 9RT
Tel: 01293 613555
Fax: 01293 613535
Website: www.novonordisk.co.uk

Owen Mumford Ltd
Brook Hill, Woodstock, Oxford OX20 1TU
Tel: 01993 812021
Fax: 01993 813466
Website: www.owenmumford.com

Pharmacia Ltd
Product Manager – Special Products, Davy Avenue, Knowhill, Milton Keynes, Bucks
MK5 8PH
Tel: 01908 661101
Fax: 01908 690091
Website: www.pnu.com

Pfizer Ltd
Ramsgate Road, Sandwich, Kent CT13 9NJ
Tel: 01304 616161
Fax: 01304 656221
Website: www.pfizer.com

Roche Diagnostics
Bell Lane, Lewes, East Sussex BN7 1LG
Tel: 01273 480444
Fax: 01273 480266
Helpline/Direct Order Line: 0800 701000
Website: www.roche.com

Servier Laboratories Ltd
Metabolism, Fulmer Hall, Windmill Road, Fulmer, Slough, Bucks SL3 6HH
Tel: 01753 662744
Fax: 01753 663456
Website: www.servier.fr

Takeda UK Ltd
Takeda House, Mercury Park, Wycombe Lane, Wooburn Green, Bucks HP10 0HH
Tel: 01628 537900
Fax: 01628 526617

Useful addresses

Diabetes-focused organisations for professionals

British Association of Retinol Screeners
Newcastle Diabetes Centre, Westgate Road, Newcastle General Hospital,
Newcastle upon Tyne NE4 6BE

Diabetes Training Centre for Primary Care Courses (Distance Learning)
Crow Trees, 27 Town Lane, Idle, Bradford BD10 8NT
Tel: 01274 617617
Fax: 01274 621621
Email: diabetestc@prestel.co.uk

Warwick Diabetes Care
University of Warwick, Coventry CV4 7AL
Tel: 024 7657 2958
Fax: 024 7657 3959
Email: diabetes@warwick.ac.uk
Website: www.diabetescare-warwick.ac.uk

A coherent point of contact for all those involved in providing diabetes care in the following ways: providing and promoting multidisciplinary diabetes education courses for health care professionals; undertaking and supporting applied diabetes research; and developing practical resources and people networks.

Other organisations for professionals

British Dietetic Association
5th Floor, Charles House,
148/9 Great Charles Street,
Queensway, Birmingham B3 3HT
Tel: 0121 200 8080
Fax: 0121 200 8081
Email: info@bda.uk.com
Website: www.bda.uk.com

English National Board for Nursing, Midwifery and Health Visiting
Victory House, 170 Tottenham Court Road
London W1P 0HA
Tel: 020 7388 3131
Fax: 020 7383 4031
Website: www.enb.org.uk

Health Development Agency
Trevelyan House, 30 Great Peter Street, London SW1P 2HW
Tel: 020 7222 5300
Fax: 020 7413 8900
Website: www.hda-online.org.uk

Health Promotion England
40 Eastbourne Terrace, London W2 3QR
Tel: 020 7725 9030
Fax: 020 7725 9031
Website: www.hpe.org.uk

Institute of Chiropodists and Podiatrists
27 Wright Street, Southport PR9 0TL
Tel: 01704 546 141
Website: www.inst-chiropodist.org.uk

A professional body the aim of which is to further the awareness of foot health issues by the general public.

Royal College of General Practitioners
14 Princes Gate, Hyde Park, London SW7 1PU
Tel: 020 7581 3232
Fax: 020 7225 3047
Email: info@rcgp.org.uk
Website: www.rcgp.org.uk

Royal Pharmaceutical Society of Great Britain
1 Lambeth High Street, London SE1 7JN
Tel: 020 7735 9141
Fax: 020 7735 7629
Email: enquiries@rpsgb.org.uk
Website: www.rpsgb.org.uk/index.html

A professional society of over 43,000 members working in all sectors of the profession, both in Britain and overseas.

Patient support organisations

Sight

Action for Blind People
14–16 Verney Road, London SE16 3DZ
Tel: 020 7635 4800
Fax: 020 7635 4900
Email: central@afbp.org
Website: www.afbp.org/homepage.htm

A national charity which aims to enable blind and partially sighted people to enjoy equal opportunities in every aspect of their lives.

Guide Dogs for the Blind Association
Burghfield Common, Reading RG7 3YG
Tel: 0870 600 2323
Email: guidedogs@guidedogs.org.uk
Website: www.gdba.org.uk

Provides guide dogs and other rehabilitation services that meet the needs of blind and partially sighted people.

Partially Sighted Society
Queens Road, Doncaster DN1 2NX
Tel: 01302 323132
Fax: 01302 368998
Email: doncaster@partsight.org.uk
Website: www.leeder.demon.co.uk/LHON/uk-pss.htm

Emphasis is placed on making the most of vision through information, advice, publications and leaflets, as well as providing information on local support groups.

Royal National Institute for the Blind
224 Great Portland Street, London W1N 5AA
Helpline: 0845 766 9999
Tel: 020 7388 1266
Fax: 020 7388 2034
Website: www.rnib.org.uk

For general information on exercise and lifestyle changes.

Hypertension/cardiac disease/stroke

British Heart Foundation
14 Fitzharding Street, London W1H 4DA
Tel: 020 7935 0185
Fax: 020 7486 5820
Website: www.bhf.org.uk

Aims to play a leading role in the fight against heart disease.

Family Heart Association
7 North Road, Maidenhead, Berkshire SL6 1PE
Tel: 01628 628 638
Fax: 01628 628 698
Email: fha@familyheart.org
Website: www.familyheart.org.uk

Stroke Association
Stroke House, 123–127 Whitecross Street, London EC1Y 8JJ
Helpline: 0845 3033 100
Email: stroke@stroke.org.uk
Website: www.stroke.org.uk

Provides support for people affected by stroke and their families.

Erectile dysfunction

Impotence Association
PO Box 10296, London SW17 9WH
Helpline: 020 8767 7791
Website: www.impotence.org.uk

A non-profit-making organisation which puts sufferers in contact with specialists around the country.

Life insurance and pensions

For information about Diabetes UK Insurance Services, send for a copy of the leaflet *Diabetes and Insurance*. Details of how to order Diabetes UK publications are given on page 290.

Diabetes UK Motor Quoteline
Tel: 01903 262900

Diabetes UK Life Assurance Quoteline
Tel: 0161 829 5600

Diabetes UK Travel Quoteline
Tel: 020 7512 0890

Devitt Insurance Services Ltd
North House
St Edwards Way
Romford, Essex RM1 3PP
Tel: 01708 355959
Fax: 0870 241 2358

Appendix IX

Template for a locally produced patient-held record card

This template has been designed by Dr Tricia Greenhalgh (GP) and Diabetes UK. If you would like further copies of this template, contact Diabetes UK. Fig. IX.1 shows the front and back of this eight-page card.

On the following pages, the template is reproduced for you to copy and adapt for your practice. For photocopying purposes, pages 8 and 1 (of the card) are on the first spread, pages 2 and 7 on the next spread, pages 6 and 3 on the third spread and pages 4 and 5 on the final spread. The guidance notes on patient-held record cards from Diabetes UK are also reproduced.

Fig. IX.1 An example of a patient-held record card. The template for this card is given on the following pages

---

What diabetes care to expect

Research has shown that people with diabetes get fewer complications, and may live longer, if they have regular check-ups, even if they do not feel ill in any way. You should agree with your doctor how often these checks should be, but at the very least, you should make sure someone examines the back of your eyes once a year. For more details, see the leaflet, 'What diabetes care to expect' available free from Diabetes UK.

Terms and tests

Blood glucose level - the amount of glucose (sugar) in the blood.
Blood pressure (BP) - the pressure level within the arteries, which indicates how hard the heart is working to pump the blood round the body.
Body mass index (BMI) - a measure of how overweight or underweight you are. A BMI above 28Kg/m means that you are seriously overweight.
Cataracts - cloudiness and thickening of the lens of the eye.
Cholesterol - a type of fat in the blood. Too much cholesterol in the blood may increase your risk of developing heart disease.
Foot pulses and sensation - checks made on the blood supply and amount of feeling in the feet.
Fructosamine - a blood test which indicates the average level of your blood glucose (sugar) during the past month.
HbA1 (or HbA1c) - a blood test which indicates the average level of your blood glucose (sugar) during the past three months.
Hyperglycaemia - high blood glucose (sugar) level.
Hypoglycaemia - low blood glucose (sugar) level.
Hyperlipidaemia - another name for high cholesterol or triglyceride levels.
Microalbuminuria - a test for very tiny amounts of protein in the urine.
Protein - urine protein is checked (with sticks) to test for damage to the kidneys. Protein is also found when there is an infection in the urine.
Retinopathy - damage to the back of the eye (retina).
Triglyceride (TG) - a type of fat in the blood.
Urea and creatinine - blood tests to check for kidney damage.
Visual acuity - an eye test which involves reading a letter chart

---

DIABETES RECORD CARD

This record card will help you receive the best care for your diabetes, and could provide vital information if you are taken ill. Please complete all the relevant details on this card, or ask the nurse or doctor to do so for you. You should bring it to all your appointments and ask the person who sees you to fill it in.

Name:_____

Address/phone:_____

_____

_____

GP name & address: _____

_____

GP phone (day): _____   (out of hours): _____

Interpreter phone: _____   Language: _____

Community pharmacist name/phone: _____

Diabetes nurse name: _____   Phone: _____

Chiropodist name: _____   Phone: _____

Hospital diabetes specialist: _____   Phone: _____

Hospital number: _____

Diabetes UK   **020 7323 1531**

Reference

Greenhalgh T (1994). Shared care for diabetes: a systematic review. *Occasional Paper 67*. London: Royal College of General Practitioners.

What diabetes care to expect

Research has shown that people with diabetes get fewer complications, and may live longer, if they have regular check-ups, **even if they do not feel ill in any way.** You should agree with your doctor how often these checks should be, but at the very least you should make sure someone examines the back of your eyes once a year. For more details, see the leaflet, What Diabetes Care to Expect, available free from Diabetes UK.

Terms and tests

Blood glucose level: the amount of glucose (sugar) in the blood.
Blood pressure (BP): the pressure level within the arteries, which indicates how hard the heart is working to pump the blood round the body.
Body mass index (BMI): a measure of how overweight or underweight you are. A BMI above 28 kg/m^2 means that you are seriously overweight.
Cataracts: cloudiness and thickening of the lens of the eye.
Cholesterol: a type of fat in the blood. Too much cholesterol in the blood may increase your risk of developing heart disease.
Hyperlipidaemia: another name for high cholesterol or triglyceride levels.
Foot pulses and sensation: checks made on the blood supply and amount of feeling in the feet.
Fructosamine: a blood test that indicates the average level of your blood glucose (sugar) during the past month.
HbA1c: a blood test that indicates the average level of your blood glucose (sugar) during the past 3 months.
Hyperglycaemia: high blood glucose (sugar) level.
Hypoglycaemia: low blood glucose (sugar) level.
Microalbuminuria: a test for very small amounts of protein in the urine.
Protein: urine protein is checked (with sticks) to test for damage to the kidneys. Protein is also found when there is an infection in the urine.
Retinopathy: damage to the back of the eye (retina).
Triglyceride (TG): a type of fat in the blood.
Urea and creatinine: blood tests to check for kidney damage.
Visual acuity: an eye test that involves reading a letter chart.

page 8

DIABETES RECORD CARD

This record card will help you to receive the best care for your diabetes, and could provide vital information if you are taken ill. Please complete all the relevant details on this card, or ask your nurse or doctor to do so for you. You should bring it to all your appointments and ask the person who sees you to fill it in.

Name .... Date of birth ....

Address ....

....

GP name & address ....

....

GP phone (day) .... (out of hours) ....

Interpreter phone .... Language ....

Community pharmacist: name/phone ....

Diabetes nurse: name .... Phone ....

Dietitian: name... Phone............................

Chiropodist: name. .... Phone............................

Hospital diabetes specialist.............................. Phone............................

Hospital number...

Diabetes UK 020 7323 1531

page 1

Medical details

Diabetes history

Date diagnosed: Weight at diagnosis:

Symptoms at diagnosis:

Family history of diabetes, blood pressure, heart disease or high cholesterol:

Initial treatment:

Past medical history

Note especially any high blood pressure, angina, heart attack or heart surgery, and stroke or similar event:

Medication

Include type and species of insulin and delivery detail if relevant:

Allergies:

page 2

Diabetes surveillance record (check-ups)

[This may be presented in a fold-out format or as several pages in a booklet; Diabetes UK recommended intervals are shown but should be modified as necessary.]

Date	3-monthly	6-monthly	3-monthly	Annual
Review control				
Weight/BMI				
Blood pressure Lying or sitting				
Standing				
Foot examination General condition				
Pulses				
Sensation				
Ankle jerks				
Urine tests Glucose				
Protein				
Microalbuminuria				
Blood tests Glucose level				
HbA1c or fructosamine				
Cholesterol				
Triglyceride				
Eye examination Fundoscopy				
Visual acuity				
Retinal photograph				

page 7

Checklist for education sessions

Below is a list of topics that you need to know about. Some are very important; the nurse or doctor should discuss them with you regularly. Some may not be relevant to you. If you are unsure, ask.

Topic	Dates discussed		
What is diabetes?			
Diet			
Tablets			
Insulin & injection technique			
Hypoglycaemia			
Hyperglycaemia			
Illness			
Blood testing			
Urine testing			
Foot care			
Importance of eye checks			
Smoking			
Alcohol			
Exercise			
Complications			
Driving/insurance			
Sexual health			
Planning pregnancy			
Diabetes UK			
Free prescriptions			
Benefits			

page 6

Personal notes and queries

This section is for you to note anything about your diabetes that you would like to discuss.

<table>
<tr><td></td></tr>
<tr><td></td></tr>
<tr><td></td></tr>
<tr><td></td></tr>
<tr><td></td></tr>
<tr><td></td></tr>
<tr><td></td></tr>
<tr><td></td></tr>
<tr><td></td></tr>
<tr><td></td></tr>
<tr><td></td></tr>
</table>

Emergencies and illnesses

Hypoglycaemic attack ('hypo'): this occurs when the blood sugar level is too low, usually when you have missed a meal or snack, or after unaccustomed exercise. It comes on SUDDENLY in a person who was not unwell. The symptoms are sweating, shaking, irritability, confusion and feeling faint. Action: TAKE SUGAR OR A SUGARY DRINK IMMEDIATELY, stop exercising and eat some long-acting carbohydrate (e.g. bread, muesli bar).

Hyperglycaemic coma: this occurs when the blood sugar level is very high. It builds up over days or weeks, so the person may have been feeling unwell for a few days. The person becomes drowsy and his or her breath may smell. Action: measure the blood glucose level with strips to confirm that it is high. Call a doctor or an ambulance. If unsure whether it is hypo- or hyper-glycaemia, give sugar anyway.

Illness: people with diabetes on insulin need MORE insulin, not less, when they are ill (e.g. with virus, 'flu, tummy bug, etc.). Even if you are eating less, DO NOT STOP YOUR INSULIN. Check the blood sugar and contact a doctor or nurse if in doubt.

page 3

Diet plan and progress record

Dietary goals:

Comments (with dates):

page 4

Chiropody/podiatry

Particular risk for foot problems:

Examinations and treatment (with dates):

page 5

Diabetes UK

Guidance on patient-held record cards

Background

Diabetes UK is often asked to provide a template for a 'standard' patient-held record card. Many patients, nurses and doctors have asked us to produce such cards centrally. Diabetes UK is reluctant to do this because we believe that all records, and particularly those that are held by patients, should be developed locally to take account of local needs and priorities. Nevertheless, we recognise that there are some general principles that should be applied in the design of patient-held records. With these in mind, we have produced the following general guidance, based on examples of existing records and advice from the Sheffield Diabetes Person Held Record Group.

Why have a patient-held record?

Patient-held records can:

- Serve as an aid to structured care (that is, help ensure that all patients get regular checks on their blood glucose control, eyes, feet, blood pressure, etc.).
- Help to educate the patient and the health professional in the principles of good diabetes care.
- Involve the patient or carer more closely in the management plan. Facilitate continuity of care when patients move house, change doctors, go on holiday, or need emergency care.

Format of the patient-held record

Most record cards we have seen are approximately A6 size (i.e. the size of a piece of A4 paper folded in half and then in half again). They usually have several pages, or come as a fold-out concertina card. The checklists for regular and annual reviews are often presented as a table, with the date down the side and items to check along the top (or vice versa). Given the wear-and-tear that a well-used record gets, a plastic or laminated cover might be sensible, and such a cover could include a slot for loose-leaf temporary additions such as letters or blood test forms.

A sample record is shown in the previous pages (pages 302–9).

What should a patient-held record contain?

This depends what the users want it to contain, which in turn will be different for particular groups of people. A child's record may look very different from an adult's. The following could be included:

1. **Patient's contact details:** name, address, emergency phone number, contact number of GP (including out-of-hours number), community pharmacist, interpreter/advocate, diabetes nurse specialist, dietitian, chiropodist and hospital consultant. For children, there should be a section on adults who 'need to know', e.g. schoolteacher. Contact details of Diabetes UK could also be given!

2. **Patient's medical and social details:** the date of diagnosis of diabetes, and how it was diagnosed (e.g. routine test, thirst, severe illness or coma, etc.). Relevant aspects of patient's medical history (especially indicators of high blood pressure or heart disease) and social or economic difficulties (e.g. housing problems, benefits received or applied for).

3. **Treatment:** details of dose and frequency of tablets or insulin. Type of insulin delivery device (e.g. make and brand of insulin 'pen'). Type of monitoring (blood or urine) and device/strips used. Other (non-diabetic) medication. Allergies.

4. **Explanatory notes:** a short section or insert box explaining to the patient why this record is important and how to use it.

5. **Instruction for emergencies:** simple, accessible instructions for the patient and carer on what to do in case of hypoglycaemic attack ('hypo'), poor control (blood glucose too high or too low), and intercurrent illness (e.g. flu, upset tummy).

6. **Education checklist:** areas for the patient and health professional to cover in education sessions. Foot care, diet review and, if relevant, pre-conception advice (for women planning a pregnancy) should be discussed at least once a year.

7. **Personal treatment plan:** a plan agreed between patient and health professional giving dietary and weight targets, advised frequency of regular check-ups, etc.

8. **Regular (3- or 6-monthly) checks:** items to be covered by the doctor or nurse at every check-up visit (see sample record).

9. **Annual review checks:** additional items to be covered once a year (see sample record).

10. **Space for patient's own notes:** 'free text' pages for patient or carer to note important symptoms or events, and questions to ask the nurse or doctor at their next consultation. Standard records often contain too little space for patient's own notes.

11. **Glossary of medical terms:** list of terms used by health professionals, with definitions (e.g. what is the HbA1c, microalbuminuria test, etc.).
12. **Detailed educational notes:** some patient-held records include sections on foot care, a standard 'diabetic diet' sheet, urine or blood testing technique, etc.

Reproduced by permission of Diabetes UK.

Index

Page numbers in *italics* indicate an illustration. Those in **bold** indicate a glossary entry.

abdominal pain 58
acarbose therapy 109
Accu-Check Advantage *136*
ACE *see* angiotensin-converting enzyme
Ace Test 51
acromegaly and diabetes 239
Actos *see* pioglitazone
acupuncture addresses 198, 199
addresses of organisations 198–200, 292–6
administrative staff role in diabetes care 11
advertising services *73*, *74*
African–Caribbeans
 cultural aspects 171–5, 182–3, 185
 ethnic origins 170
 incidence of diabetes in UK 25
albumin excretion 245
Albustix 51
alcohol consumption 97
 in ethnic populations 173
 information to patients 204
alimentary tract dysfunction 249
alpha-blocker therapy for hypertension 89
alpha cells **xxv**
alpha-glucosidase inhibitor therapy 109
Amaryl *see* glimepiride
amino acid derivative therapy 105–6
amyotrophy, diabetic **xxv**

angina patients 89
angiotensin II receptor antagonists
 therapy for hypertension 89
angiotensin-converting enzyme (ACE)
 inhibitors for hypertension 89, 252
 and diabetic nephropathy 246
 side effects 252
Aretaeus 224
aromatherapy addresses 198, 199
Asians
 cultural aspects 171–5, 185
 ethnic origins 170
 incidence of diabetes 24, 170–1
 see also specific religions
aspirin therapy 89, 254–5
atherosclerosis risks 253
attitude problems and diabetes 189
audit and evaluation of general
 practice diabetes care 215–20
 outcome measures 217–18
 process measures 216
Audit Commission Report 2000
 (*Testing Times*) xxiii, 29
Autolet 51
Avandia *see* rosiglitazone

Baisakhi-Sikhs festival 180
Balance for Beginners 291
Band 3 level reimbursement 3
Banting, Frederick 224
basement membrane thickening 243
bathing habits in ethnic populations 173
BDA *see* Diabetes UK

resources 287–8
self-monitoring 132–7
team, expectations from 272–3
    role 30–5, 273–4
    members 272
    see also general practice diabetes
      care system
caste system in Hindus 177
cataracts 146, 149, 249
causes of diabetes, secondary 239–42
celebrations, information to patients
    about 204
cereals 99, 184
cervical screening, information to
    patients 207
Chanucah festival 181
check-up card 305
Chevraul 224
children
    care team 31
    clinics 30
    diagnosis 269
    incidence of diabetes in UK 23
    information to patients 208
    retinopathy in 248
    St Vincent Declaration 269–70
    treatment 269
chiropodist **xxv**
    referral to 167
    role 33–4
chiropody **xxv**, 33
    card 309
    information to patients 205
    services links 71
chocolate 97
cholesterol levels 255
    screening 253
cigarette smoking in ethnic
    populations 172–3
circulatory problems causing diabetic
    foot 156, *157*
classification of diabetes xx, xxi,
    233–4, 235

clerical staff role in diabetes care 11
clinical audit 215–20
clinical governance xxii–xxiii
clinics 30
    essential equipment 49–53
    foot 167
    materials and resources 53–6
    requirements 49
    see also general practice diabetes
      care system
Clinistix 51
clock/wristwatch 50
coma xxv, **xxvi**
combination therapy 110–11
communication
    with ethnic populations 171
    problems 171, 189
community nurse
    diabetic courses 16–17
    role in diabetes care 9
complementary therapies addresses
    198–200
complications in diabetes 243–57
    fear of 188
    markers audit 217
    prevention strategy 88–90
consequences of diabetes 25–6
contact lens fitter 147
contraceptive pill and diabetes 240
convenience foods 100
cooperation card 48
coordination of care provision 6
corns 164
coronary heart disease risk factors 252
corticosteroid therapy and diabetes
    240
cost of diabetes 27–8
cotton wool/tissues 50, 119
counsellor role in diabetes care 9
courses on diabetes 15–16
culture aspects and diabetes 169–86,
    188
Cushing's syndrome and diabetes 239

hearty breakfast test 63–4
heat and foot care 164
height gauge 50
herbal medicine 185
  addresses 198, 199
hereditary causes of diabetes 241
Hinduism 175–7
history of diabetes mellitus 223–6
history taking, cultural differences 175
Holi festival 177
holidays, information to patients 211
homoeopathy addresses 199, 200
honeymoon period **xxvi**
hooka smoking 172
hormonal causes of diabetes 239
hormone replacement therapy,
    information to patients 207
hospital
  foot care 155
  referral criteria 79
  referral for feet 167
house-bound patients 46, 66
human insulin **xxvi**, 113, 122
  changing to 115
hunger 58
hyperfiltration 245
hyperglycaemia **xxvi**, 126
  causes 126–7
  diagnosis 228
  in Hindus 177
  information to patients 203
  prevention 127
  symptoms 127
hypertension
  control 89, 251–2
  and diabetic nephropathy 246
  incidence 253
  microalbuminaemia and 82
  support organisations 299–300
Hypertension Optimal Treatment
    (HOT) Study xxi, 261
hypnotherapy addresses 198, 199
hypo *see* hypoglycaemia

hypoglycaemia 130–1
  carbohydrates for 95
  causes 130
  diagnosis 227
  diminished warning signs 130
  driving and 211
  emergency treatment needs 53
  from glibenclamide 103
  prevention 114–15, 121
  treatment 121–2, 131
hypoglycaemic agents **xxvi**, 233
  information to patients 202
  research history 225
Hypostop gel **xxvi**

IDDM *see* type 1 diabetes
identification cards 53
IFG *see* impaired fasting glycaemia
IGT *see* impaired glucose tolerance
illness and diabetes, guidelines for
    management 127–8
illness rules, information to patients
    203
immunisations, information to
    patients 208, 212
impaired fasting glycaemia (IFG) **xxvi**,
    64, 235–6
impaired glucose tolerance (IGT)
    xxvi, 64, 235
  gestational 236
impotence 250
incidence of diabetes xx, **xxvi**
  in ethnic populations 70–1
  in UK 23–5
incontinence 58
indapamide therapy for hypertension
    89
indemnity for practice nurses 4
Indian populations, diabetic
    nephropathy and 245
Indo-Asian populations, incidence of
    diabetes 170–1
infections 58, 59

influenza immunisation, information to patients 208
information
  booklets/leaflets 53
  contact number need 122
  foot care 163–6
  getting message across 192–3
  links and contact numbers 53–4, 69–73
  needs and problems in diabetes 189–90
  organisation and recording 54
  technology 192–3
injections
  bleeding after 123
  care of equipment 121
  dummy 118
  equipment 118–19
  forgetting 122
  giving 120
  sites 113, 114, 120
insulin 110–23
  analogues 116
  benefits 118
  bottle/cartridge 118
  changing species 115
  coma *see* coma
  delivery devices 113–14, 115
  dose 114, 116
  drawing up 119
  facts about 113–14
  hypoglycaemic action *116*
  onset/rise/peak/ fall/duration of action 114, 115–16
  pens **xxvi**, 113–14
  reactions 114
  research history 225
  resistance 251
  self-administration 116–17
  side effect management 114–15
  sources/species 113, 115
  therapy for type 2 diabetes 111–13, 233

  care team role 274
  diabetes 233
  with drug therapy 110–11
  information to patients 202–3
  trial 112
  type 114, 115–16
  wrong dose 122–3
  see also specific types of insulin, e.g. beef insulin; injections
insulinomas 241
insurance companies 210, 211, 300
integrated care 48–9
intermediate-acting insulin **xxvii**, 114
International Consensus Standards of Practice for Diabetes Education 187
interviewing, motivational 190
intraocular pressure measurement 149
iron metabolism abnormality and diabetes 240
irritability 58, 59
ischaemic foot 159
Islam 178–9
islet cell
  transplants 261
  tumours and diabetes 240–1
islets of Langerhans **xxvii**
isophane **xxvii**, 114

Jainism 177
Joint British Diabetes Association xiii
Journal of Diabetes Nursing 292
journals 291
Judaism 180–1
juvenile-onset diabetes *see* type 1 diabetes

ketoacidosis **xxvii**, 114
  mortality 27
ketonuria **xxvii**, 58
  testing equipment 51
Ketostix 51
Ketur Test 51

patient
education (contd)
for self-monitoring 132–7
session checklist 306
identification, importance 122
records *see* person care record
card
responsibilities 275
satisfaction audit 218
PCDUK *see* Primary Care Diabetes UK
pen *see* insulin pens
pensions, addresses 300
peripheral neuropathy *see*
neuropathy, peripheral
peripheral vascular disease mortality
27
person care record card 48, 54–6, *55*,
86, 301–12
pharmacist role in diabetes care 10
physician role in diabetes care 31
pinhole card 52
pioglitazone therapy 107, 108, 110
plasma glucose level tests 63, 64, 65–6
pneumococcal immunisation,
information to patients 208
podiatrist *see* chiropodist
podiatry *see* chiropody
polyuria **xxvii**, 58
Poole Study xxi, 259–60
porcine insulin **xxvii**, 113, 225
changing from 114
Islam and 178
Judaism and
posters 53, 59, *60*, 67, 72, *142*, 291
post-myocardial patients 89
postprandial glucose regulator
therapy (PPGRs) **xxvii**, 89,
104–5, 108
Practical Diabetes International 292
practice manager role in diabetes care
11
practice nurse role in diabetes care
4–8, 46

pravastatin therapy 89
pre-conception counselling 206, 228
pregnancy and diabetes 236–7
counselling 228
information to patients 206
outcome audit 217
Prevalence and Incidence of Type 2
Diabetes (Poole Study) xxi,
259–60
prevalence of diabetes xx, **xxvii**
in ethnic populations 170–1
type 1 228
type 2 231
in UK 23–5
worldwide 170
prevention 231
primary care
changes in NHS xxii
provision 284–6
team, books for 288–9
self-help 18
education needs 19–21
see also care team
Primary Care Diabetes – a National
Enquiry xxii, 260
professional education requirements
16–17
protein
restriction in diet 246
testing equipment 50, 51
proteinuria **xxvii**, 245
screening 82
psychiatric team role in diabetes care 9
psychotherapist role in diabetes care 9
public awareness of diabetes 59–60
pulses 99, 184
Purim festival 181

quality of life audit 218

racial variations 24–5
Ramadan festival 179
ramipril therapy 89

spices and condiments 184
sports, information to patients 209
St Vincent Declaration on Diabetes
    xiii–xv, 215–16
    Diabetes Care and Research in
        Europe 267–8
    recommendations for the care of
        children 269–70
St Vincent Joint Task Force Subgroup
    Report on Training and
    Professional Development in
    Diabetes Care 15
Starlix *see* nateglinide
statistics on diabetes xx, 30, 259–62
statutory rights 271
stick tests for microalbuminuria 245,
    246
stockings 160, *163*, 166
strips 50, 51, 52, 137
stroke
    mortality 27
    support organisations 299–300
sugar intake in diet 93, 94, 97
Sukkot festival 181
sulphonylureas therapy **xxvii**, 88–9,
    102–2, 108
    in combination 110
    research history 225
support organisations 298–300
Supreme 51
surveillance card 305
sweet foods 95, 100
symptoms of diabetes mellitus 57–60
    relief aims 87
syringes 118–19

Task Force for Diabetes xiii-xiv
team care
    educational needs 13–21
    provision 3–12, 46–7
    role 30–1
    see also general practice diabetes
        care system

technology used in diabetes care, new
    xxii
telling the patient 63
tests to be expected 302
tetanus immunisation, information to
    patients 208
thiazide therapy and diabetes 240
    side effects 252
thiazolidinedione therapy **xxvii**, 88–9,
    106–7, 108, 109, 251
    in combination 110
thirst 58
thrush infections 58
thyroxine therapy and diabetes 240
tights 160, *163*, 166
tingling 58
tiredness 58, 59
toenail care 164
toilet habits in ethnic populations 173
Tolanase *see* tolazamide
tolazamide 102
tolbutamide therapy 102, 103, 108
travel, information to patients 211,
    212
treatment for diabetes 87–100
    aims 87–8
    effectiveness 28–9
    in children 269
    new xxii
    strategy 88–90
    see also under type 1 *and* type 2
        diabetes *and specific therapies*
triglyceride levels 255
tumours, hormonal, and diabetes 239
tuning fork 52
type 1 diabetes **xxvii**, 227–9
    causes 228–9
    complications 243
    diagnosis 227–8, 232
    incidence in UK 23
    microalbuminaemia screening
        82–3
    prevalence 228

**Have you found *Providing Diabetes Care in General Practice*
useful and practical? If so, you may be interested in other
books from Class Publishing:**

Vital Diabetes (2nd edition)   £14.99
Charles Fox BM, FRCP and Mary MacKinnon MMedSci, RGN

Managing diabetes in your practice is a superhuman task – especially with
treatment guidelines changing all the time. This handy reference guide is here to
help.
> *Vital Diabetes* gives you:

- Clear and concise information at a glance;
- The confidence to know that your patients are getting the best advice on
  treatment and self-care;
- Patient (and carer) information you can photocopy for patients to take
  away with them whenever they need it;
- All the vital facts and figures about diabetes, for your information and use.

Diabetes in the real world   £19.95
Charles Fox BM, FRCP and Anthony Pickering BM, BCH

Charles Fox and Tony Pickering confront the issues and problems of diabetes
care in general practice, from the prospective of the GP. This is the real world,
inhabited by real people, and by GPs with limited resources and a desperate
shortage of time – rather than the artificially ordered environment of the
textbook. This practical handbook will increase your confidence in dealing with
the varied needs of all people with diabetes in general practice – whether young
or old, type 1 or type 2, healthy or sick.

CancerBACUP directory of cancer services   £19.99

CancerBACUP is the UK's leading cancer information charity, and this directory
contains information about key resources for cancer patients and their families,
as well as information written specifically for health professionals. It includes
comprehensive details of national and local organizations and support groups,
all UK hospices, a guide to patient information, CancerBACUP's statements on
controversial cancer topics and information on UK treatment guidelines.

COPD in Primary Care

£24.99

David Bellamy MBE, BSc, FRCP, MRCGP, DRCOG
and Rachel Booker RGN HV

Chronic Obstructive Pulmonary Disease (the spectrum of diseases including chronic bronchitis, emphysema, long-standing irreversible asthma and small airways disease) is one of the most common and important respiratory disorders seen in primary care. This clear and helpful resource manual addresses the management requirements of GPs and practice nurses. In this book, you will find guidance, protocols, plans and tests – all appropriate to the primary care situation – that will streamline your diagnosis and management of COPD. It focuses on the five goals for COPD management laid out by the British Thoracic Society:

- Early and accurate diagnosis;
- Best control of symptoms;
- Prevention of deterioration;
- Prevention of complications;
- Improved quality of life.

This manual is produced in conjunction with *The National Asthma and Respiratory Training Centre* and endorsed by the *GPs in Asthma Group*.

The 'at your fingertips' series

Our series, named *'at your fingertips'*, seeks to help those who, having been diagnosed with a condition, have countless questions that need answering. All our authors are medical experts, at the top of their profession.

The formula for the series follows a question-and-answer format, with real questions from sufferers and their families answered by medical, nursing and welfare experts. We sell tens of thousands of books each year.

"Woe betide any clinicians or nurses whose patients have read this invaluable source of down-to-earth information when they have not." – *The Lancet*

And at only £14.99 plus £3 p&p each – with a full money-back guarantee – what have you got to lose?!

Allergies at your fingertips
  Dr Joanne Clough
Asthma at your fingertips
  Dr Mark Levy, Professor Sean Hilton and Greta Barnes
Cancer at your fingertips
  Val Speechley and Max Rosenfield
Dementia at your fingertips
  Harry Cayton, Professor Nori Graham and Dr James Warner
Diabetes at your fingertips
  Professor Peter Sonksen, Dr Charles Fox and Sue Judd
Epilepsy at your fingertips
  Brian Chappell and Professor Pam Crawford
Heart health at your fingertips
  Dr Graham Jackson
High blood pressure at your fingertips
  Dr Julian Tudor Hart and Dr Tom Fahey
Kidneys at your fingertips
  Dr Andy Stein and Janet Wild
Multiple sclerosis at your fingertips
  Dr Ian Robinson, Dr Stuart Neilson, Dr Frank Clifford Rose
Motor neurone disease at your fingertips
  Dr Stuart Neilson and Dr Ian Robinson
Parkinson's at your fingertips
  Dr Marie Oxtoby and Professor Adrian Williams
Psoriasis at your fingertips
  Dr Tim Mitchell and Rebecca Penzer
Sex at your fingertips
  Philip Kell and Vanessa Griffiths
Stroke at your fingertips
  Dr Anthony Rudd, Penny Irwin and Bridget Penhale

PRIORITY ORDER FORM

Cut out or photocopy this form and send it (post free in the UK) to:
Class Publishing Priority Service,
FREEPOST (PAM 6219), Plymouth PL6 7ZZ
Fax (01752) 202333

Please send me urgently   Price per copy
(tick boxes below)   postage included (*UK only*)

☐ **Providing diabetes care in general practice**	£27.99
☐ **Vital diabetes**	£17.99
☐ **Diabetes in the real world**	£22.95
☐ **CancerBACUP directory of cancer services**	£22.99
☐ **COPD in primary care**	£27.99
☐ **Allergies at your fingertips**	£17.99
☐ **Asthma at your fingertips**	£17.99
☐ **Cancer at your fingertips**	£17.99
☐ **Dementia at your fingertips**	£17.99
☐ **Diabetes at your fingertips**	£17.99
☐ **Epilepsy at your fingertips**	£17.99
☐ **Heart health at your fingertips**	£17.99
☐ **High blood pressure at your fingertips**	£17.99
☐ **Kidneys at your fingertips**	£17.99
☐ **Multiple sclerosis at your fingertips**	£17.99
☐ **Motor neurone disease at your fingertips**	£17.99
☐ **Parkinson's at your fingertips**	£17.99
☐ **Psoriasis at your fingertips**	£17.99
☐ **Sex at your fingertips**	£17.99
☐ **Stroke at your fingertips**	£17.99
	TOTAL _____

Easy ways to pay

Cheque: I enclose a cheque payable to Class Publishing for £_____

Credit card: Please debit my ☐ Access ☐ Visa ☐ Amex ☐ Switch

Number ☐☐☐☐☐☐☐☐☐☐☐☐☐☐☐☐   Expiry date ____/____

Name ....

My address for delivery is ....

Town .... County .... Postcode ....

Telephone number (*in case of query*) ....

Credit card billing address if different from above ....

Town .... County .... Postcode ....

Class Publishing's guarantee: remember that if, for any reason, you are not satisfied with these books, we will refund all your money, without any questions asked. Prices and VAT rates may be altered for reasons beyond our control.

☐ Please do not send me details of other Class Publishing books.